Food Bioactives: Impact on Brain and Cardiometabolic Health—Findings from In Vitro to Human Studies

Food Bioactives: Impact on Brain and Cardiometabolic Health—Findings from In Vitro to Human Studies

Editors

Nenad Naumovski
Domenico Sergi

MDPI • Basel • Beijing • Wuhan • Barcelona • Belgrade • Manchester • Tokyo • Cluj • Tianjin

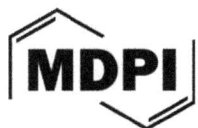

Editors

Nenad Naumovski
School of Rehabilitation and
Exercise Sciences,
Faculty of Health,
University of Canberra
Australia

Domenico Sergi
Department of Translational
Medicine and for Romagna,
University of Ferrara
Italy

Editorial Office
MDPI
St. Alban-Anlage 66
4052 Basel, Switzerland

This is a reprint of articles from the Special Issue published online in the open access journal *Foods* (ISSN 2304-8158) (available at: https://www.mdpi.com/journal/foods/special_issues/Food_Bioactives_Cardiometabolic_Implications).

For citation purposes, cite each article independently as indicated on the article page online and as indicated below:

LastName, A.A.; LastName, B.B.; LastName, C.C. Article Title. *Journal Name* **Year**, *Volume Number*, Page Range.

ISBN 978-3-0365-4041-2 (Hbk)
ISBN 978-3-0365-4042-9 (PDF)

© 2022 by the authors. Articles in this book are Open Access and distributed under the Creative Commons Attribution (CC BY) license, which allows users to download, copy and build upon published articles, as long as the author and publisher are properly credited, which ensures maximum dissemination and a wider impact of our publications.

The book as a whole is distributed by MDPI under the terms and conditions of the Creative Commons license CC BY-NC-ND.

Contents

About the Editors vii

Nenad Naumovski and Domenico Sergi
Food Bioactives: Impact on Brain and Cardiometabolic Health—Findings from In Vitro to Human Studies
Reprinted from: *Foods* 2021, 10, 1045, doi:10.3390/foods10051045 1

Domenico Sergi, Alex Gélinas, Jimmy Beaulieu, Justine Renaud, Emilie Tardif-Pellerin, Jérôme Guillard and Maria-Grazia Martinoli
Anti-Apoptotic and Anti-Inflammatory Role of Trans ε-Viniferin in a Neuron–Glia Co-Culture Cellular Model of Parkinson's Disease
Reprinted from: *Foods* 2021, 10, 586, doi:10.3390/foods10030586 5

Fernando Leal-Martínez, Denise Franco, Andrea Peña-Ruiz, Fabiola Castro-Silva, Andrea A. Escudero-Espinosa, Oscar G. Rolón-Lacarrier, Mardia López-Alarcón, Ximena De León, Mariana Linares-Eslava and Antonio Ibarra
Effect of a Nutritional Support System (Diet and Supplements) for Improving Gross Motor Function in Cerebral Palsy: An Exploratory Randomized Controlled Clinical Trial
Reprinted from: *Foods* 2020, 9, 1449, doi:10.3390/foods9101449 19

Jackson Williams, Andrew J. McKune, Ekavi N. Georgousopoulou, Jane Kellett, Nathan M. D'Cunha, Domenico Sergi, Duane Mellor and Nenad Naumovski
The Effect of L-Theanine Incorporated in a Functional Food Product (Mango Sorbet) on Physiological Responses in Healthy Males: A Pilot Randomised Controlled Trial
Reprinted from: *Foods* 2020, 9, 371, doi:10.3390/foods9030371 35

Manja M. Zec, Aletta E. Schutte, Cristian Ricci, Jeannine Baumgartner, Iolanthe M. Kruger and Cornelius M. Smuts
Long-Chain Polyunsaturated Fatty Acids Are Associated with Blood Pressure and Hypertension over 10-Years in Black South African Adults Undergoing Nutritional Transition
Reprinted from: *Foods* 2019, 8, 394, doi:10.3390/foods8090394 49

Mikkel R. Deutch, Daniela Grimm, Markus Wehland, Manfred Infanger and Marcus Krüger
Bioactive Candy: Effects of Licorice on the Cardiovascular System
Reprinted from: *Foods* 2019, 8, 495, doi:10.3390/foods8100495 65

About the Editors

Nenad Naumovski

Nedad Naumovskiis a food scientist and molecular nutritionist and works at the University of Canberra (ACT, Australia) as Associate Professor in Food Science and Human Nutrition. He leads a Functional Foods and Nutrition Research Laboratory (FFNR Laboratory) and holds academic conjoint positions as the Visiting Professor at the Harokopio University of Athens (Athens, Greece) and University of Newcastle (NSW, Australia). He has presented the findings of his research group at several academic and scientific societies as an invited guest speaker and provided number of plenary talks including prestigious Australian Academy of Science. Dr Naumovski has a strong research interest in the development of functional foods and the effects of food and nutrients on psycho-cardiological markers associated with healthy ageing. Currently, he leads several projects relating to the flavor augmentation and consumption of different plant bioactives on the reduction of stress and anxiety, improvements in focus, attention and quality of sleep.

Domenico Sergi

Domenico Sergi is a nutrition scientist with a PhD in Human Nutrition pursued at the Rowett Institute (University of Aberdeen, UK) in 2016 under the supervision of Prof. Lynda M. Williams, Dr Janice Drew, Dr Iain Greig and Dr James Hislop. In February 2017 he moved to Maastricht where he was appointed as a postdoctoral researcher within the Diabetes and Metabolism Research Group (University of Maastricht) to study the effect of pharmacological and nutritional compounds on insulin sensitivity, substrate metabolism and mitochondrial function in human primary myocytes and skeletal muscle cell lines. In September 2017 he moved to Adelaide (Sounth Australian Health and Medical Research Institute) where he was appointed as a postdoctoral research fellow at the Commonwealth Scientific and Industrial Research Organisation (CSIRO) to investigate novel approaches in nutrition for health. After which he moved to Canada to start his first tenure-track position as a professor in the department of medical biology at the "Université du Québec à Trois-Rivières". Domenico now holds a tenure-track position (RTDb) in Nutrition and Dietetics in the Department of Translational Medicine at University of Ferrara (Italy). Domenico is interested in the tight relationship between nutrition and health and how nutrients and specific dietary patterns can affect human health, with particular focus upon metabolic health. His main interest lies in the mechanisms underpinning the development of obesity and its comorbidities, with a particular focus on metabolic inflammation and lipotoxicity.

Editorial

Food Bioactives: Impact on Brain and Cardiometabolic Health—Findings from In Vitro to Human Studies

Nenad Naumovski [1,2,3,*] and Domenico Sergi [4,5]

1. Discipline of Nutrition and Dietetics, Faculty of Health, University of Canberra, Canberra, ACT 2601, Australia
2. Functional Foods and Nutrition Research (FFNR) Laboratory, University of Canberra, Bruce, ACT 2617, Australia
3. Discipline of Nutrition-Dietetics, School of Health Science and Education, Harokopio University, 17671 Athens, Greece
4. Molecular Nutrition, Department of Medical Biology, Université du Québec à Trois-Rivières, Trois-Rivières, QC G8Z 4M3, Canada; Domenico.sergi2@uqtr.ca or d.88@live.it
5. Adelaide Medical School, The University of Adelaide, Adelaide, SA 5000, Australia
* Correspondence: Nenad.naumovski@canberra.edu.au; Tel.: +61-2-6206-8719

Modern society is currently (and probably more than ever) immersed in the changing concept of food, seeking the beneficial functions of foods rather than only as a mean to quench hunger and support basic nutritional needs. In this context, we are facing a change in the expectations that consumers have from food items, accompanied by an increased attention towards food bioactive derivatives with health boosting properties. These emerging perceptions of food as a key discriminant in human health are fueled by the already strong evidence linking unhealthy dietary patterns with the onset and progression of several chronic diseases, ranging from type 2 diabetes mellitus (T2DM) to cancer and neurodegenerative diseases. On the contrary, functional foods and their bioactive components may represent a nutritional cornerstone to improve the quality of diet and ameliorate or prevent (in some cases) nutrition-related diseases. Bioactives are unlike pharmaceuticals (compounds used to alleviate symptoms and cure disease). Nevertheless, the latest findings indicate that the clear gap between the two products (bioactives and pharmaceuticals) is becoming narrower and in some cases, they are becoming interchangeable.

In agreement with the aforementioned considerations, the interest of the general population with respect to functional foods containing bioactive molecules is in constant expansion, which provides an impetus for research in this field. Indeed, several studies, including in vitro investigations, clinical trials and observational studies related to food and dietary patterns have already identified, proposed and in some cases, challenged the mechanisms of action of food bioactive derivatives. Therefore, the main aim of this Special Issue was to provide an opportunity to bring together high-quality manuscripts that showcase the current knowledge in relation to food bioactives and their impact on brain and cardiometabolic health.

The article by Deutch et al. (2019) is a comprehensive work identifying the compositional properties of licorice and the potential impacts on blood pressure and the cardiovascular system [1]. Licorice is the root of the legume *Glycyrrhiza glabra* that is commonly grown in warm climatic areas such as the Middle East, Asia and southern parts of Europe. For several millennia, this root was used in traditional medicines of many countries as an ailment for a number of different diseases and heath conditions, such as gastrointestinal symptoms and respiratory diseases. Nowadays, a broad-spectrum of health-related properties have been ascribed to licorice, including immunostimulatory effects; anti-ulcer, anti-cancer, anti-viral and anti-microbial effects; in addition to the protection of the nervous and cardiovascular systems. Although licorice consists of over 300 potential bioactive compounds, the authors report that the health effects elicited by licorice mainly rely on the bioactive glycyrrhizin. This molecule is a prodrug that is converted into 3β-monoglucuronyl-18β-glycerrhetinic acid (3MGA) and 18β-glycerrhetinic acid (GA) in the small intestine. Despite both compounds having been associated with a variety of potential health benefits, 3MGA and GA can also inhibit the hydroxysteroid dehydrogenase II enzyme, which is responsible for oxidizing cortisol into cortisone. Therefore, high licorice consumption can also potentially promote hypernatremia, hypokalemia and fluid volume retention. Furthermore, the authors report on the findings from a relatively recent meta-analysis where the increased intake of licorice was associated with significant increases in systolic (5.45 mmHg) and diastolic (3.19 mmHg) blood pressures (BPs). The authors also propose caution against the consumption of large quantities of licorice as some negative health effects may occur.

The incidence and occurrence of neurodegenerative diseases is on a constant increase worldwide, with Alzheimer's Disease (AD) and Parkinson's Disease (PD) being the most prevalent. A pivotal pathophysiological aspect of these diseases is the progressive neuronal loss that can be triggered by oxidative stress, mitochondrial dysfunction and neuroinflammation. In this regard, strategies aimed at counteracting the damaging effects of oxidative stress and neuroinflammation are considered as promising avenues to prevent neurodegeneration. In this context, bioactive molecules may play a role in counteracting the pathophysiological mechanisms linked with neurodegeneration. Of these, ε-viniferin (resveratrol dimer), as reported in the paper by Sergi et al., has shown to share similar effects with resveratrol in relation to neuroprotection in animal models of AD and Huntington's Disease [2]. Nevertheless, the effects of ε-viniferin on oxidative stress and inflammation-induced injury in dopaminegeric neurons remain relatively unexplored. In this study, the authors reported the neuroprotective potential of ε-viniferin in nerve growth factor (NGF)-differentiated PC12 cells, an in vitro dopaminergic model of Parkinson's disease (PD), and assessed the potential anti-inflammatory properties of this nutraceutical in a N9 microglia-neuronal PC12 cell co-culture system. The cells were pretreated with ε-viniferin, resveratrol and their mixtures before the administration of 6-hydroxydompamine (6-OHDA) that is recognized for inducing PD-like symptoms in animal models. In addition, the authors also investigated the effects of these stilbenes on the potential reduction in lipopolysaccharide-induced inflammation. The findings indicated that ε-viniferin alone or in combination with resveratrol protects the neuronal dopaminergic PC12 cells from 6-OHDA-induced cytotoxicity and apoptosis as well as the neuronal cytotoxicity triggered by microglial activation.

L-Theanine (L-THE) is the most abundant non-proteinogenic amino acid found in green tea. Its consumption has been proposed to be associated with stress-reducing effects and antihypertensive properties as well as improvements in cognitive functioning. In consideration of this, and given the recent commercial availability of relatively pure L-THE, there is a strong potential for the development of functional food products that contain this amino acid as a bioactive ingredient. A study by Williams et al. (2020) investigated the physiological responses, including heart rate (HR), heart rate variability (HRV) and BP in healthy males (n = 11), following the acute ingestion of a functional food products (mango sorbet) containing 200 mg of pure L-THE [3]. In this double blind, placebo-controlled cross-over trial, the participants were required to consume the test food or placebo mango sorbet (color and flavor matched) after which their physiological responses were continuously monitored over a period of 90 min. The study reported no significant differences between the intervention and placebo or within the individual groups (all p's > 0.05). Furthermore, the results of this study indicate that there was also no parasympathetic response following L-THE intake (determined via the HR response). The authors have proposed that these findings could potentially be due to the interaction between L-THE and the food matrix it was embedded in, which may have affected L-THE bioavailability. In addition, the authors have acknowledged the limitations of the study, such as the sample size (considering this being the pilot trial) and the selection of healthy participants. Nevertheless, this study highlights the importance of the careful selection of the food matrix composition in the development of future functional foods containing L-THE as an active ingredient, particularly considering that the matrix itself may affect the bioavailability of bioactive molecules.

The urbanization of sub-Saharan Africa is associated with a dietary shift towards the overconsumption of energy-dense foods, which in turn significantly contributes to the overall increase in cardiovascular disease, obesity and type 2 diabetes observed in this geographical area. A study by Zec et al. (2019) investigated the South African cohort of the Prospective Urban Rural Epidemiology (PURE) study, an international study investigating the health complications associated with urbanization in *low-*, *middle-* and *high*-income countries [4]. In this study, the authors examined data from 300 adults (older than 30 years of age) on the occurrence of hypertension and long-chain polyunsaturated fatty acids (PUFA) status. Data were analyzed from three consecutive examinations (2005, 2010 and 2015). The results revealed that the ten-year hypertension incidence significantly increased among rural participants (+20%, $p = 0.001$) while there was no significant change in urban participants ($p = 0.253$). Moreover, regardless of urbanization, n-6 PUFA status increased while the eicosapentanoic acid (EPA) status decreased over the 10-year period. Furthermore, authors reported an increase in BP (+2.92 systolic and +1.94 mmHg diastolic) and 1.46 higher odds of being hypertensive in the participants in the highest EPA tertile. In black South Africans included in this study sample, individual plasma n-6 PUFA were inversely associated with BP while EPA was associated with increases in BP leading to hypertension. Nonetheless, these findings should be interpreted with caution, especially in consideration of the well-documented positive effects of omega-3 fatty acids, such as EPA, on cardiovascular health.

The study by Leal-Martinez et al. (2020) is an exploratory randomized controlled clinical trial investigating the effects of a nutritional support system for improving motor function in children living with cerebral palsy (CP) in Mexico [5]. CP is one of the most common disabilities in childhood and changes to gross motor function is one of the main characteristics associated with this disease that can contribute to malnutrition in patients with CP. Furthermore, parasitosis is very common in this population sample and can contribute to the impairment of nutrient absorption. In this study, children with CP ($n = 30$) were divided in the three groups ($n = 10$ each): follow-up (monitoring of the diet only), control (dewormed and received nutritional therapy recommended by WHO) and intervention group (dewormed and received nutritional support system (diet and supplements)). All participants received Bobath physical therapy. The supplemental composition included a combination of amino acids (glutamine and arginine), vitamins (folic acid, cholecalciferol, ascorbic acid, nicotinic acid), minerals (zinc and selenium), spirulina, vegetable-based protein and n-3 PUFA. In addition, the participants also consumed probiotics (200 mg of *Saccharomyces Bouladii*) every 12 h for three days in the basal period and at week 7 for correcting malabsorption. The overall findings of the study were that a nutritional intervention consisting of diet and combination of supplements resulted in an improvement in gross motor function and promoted increases in walking ability in children living with CP.

In summary, the field of food bioactives is exceptionally diverse and it is a rapidly growing area of research and development. This is also fueled by the availability of novel analytical techniques, experimental models of human disease, and by an increase in consumer demand, seeking food products supported by solid health claims. Indeed, in order to meet these expectations, there is an ever-increasing need to translate the discoveries related to the health-promoting effects of food bioactives from the bench to the clinic, particularly in relation to brain and cardiometabolic health which represent areas of research with the greatest potential impact of human health. The findings reported in the studies published as part of this Special Issue further confirm the potential beneficial role of food bioactive derivatives and pave the way for future investigations aimed at further dissecting the impact of food bioactive molecules on human health. Nevertheless, we must not overlook the fact that food bioactives should not be considered as a panacea in the battle against human chronic diseases, as their health promoting effects cannot be sustained or even occur in the absence of a healthy lifestyle characterized by adherence to healthy dietary patterns and physical activity. We (the co-editors of this Special Issue) are thankful to the authors and reviewers who have contributed to this issue by sharing their knowledge, findings and time.

Author Contributions: N.N. and D.S. wrote the paper. All authors have read and agreed to the published version of the manuscript.

Funding: This research received no external funding.

Conflicts of Interest: The authors declare no conflict of interest.

References

1. Deutch, M.R.; Grimm, D.; Wehland, M.; Infanger, M.; Kruger, M. Bioactive Candy: Effects of Licorice on the Cardiovascular System. *Foods* **2019**, *8*, 495. [CrossRef] [PubMed]
2. Sergi, D.; Gelinas, A.; Beaulieu, J.; Renaud, J.; Tardif-Pellerin, E.; Guillard, J.; Martinoli, M.G. Anti-Apoptotic and Anti-Inflammatory Role of Trans epsilon-Viniferin in a Neuron-Glia Co-Culture Cellular Model of Parkinson's Disease. *Foods* **2021**, *10*, 586. [CrossRef] [PubMed]
3. Williams, J.; McKune, A.J.; Georgousopoulou, E.N.; Kellett, J.; D'Cunha, N.M.; Sergi, D.; Mellor, D.; Naumovski, N. The Effect of L-Theanine Incorporated in a Functional Food Product (Mango Sorbet) on Physiological Responses in Healthy Males: A Pilot Randomised Controlled Trial. *Foods* **2020**, *9*, 371. [CrossRef] [PubMed]
4. Zec, M.M.; Schutte, A.E.; Ricci, C.; Baumgartner, J.; Kruger, I.M.; Smuts, C.M. Long-Chain Polyunsaturated Fatty Acids Are Associated with Blood Pressure and Hypertension over 10-Years in Black South African Adults Undergoing Nutritional Transition. *Foods* **2019**, *8*, 394. [CrossRef] [PubMed]
5. Leal-Martinez, F.; Franco, D.; Pena-Ruiz, A.; Castro-Silva, F.; Escudero-Espinosa, A.A.; Rolon-Lacarrier, O.G.; Lopez-Alarcon, M.; De Leon, X.; Linares-Eslava, M.; Ibarra, A. Effect of a Nutritional Support System (Diet and Supplements) for Improving Gross Motor Function in Cerebral Palsy: An Exploratory Randomized Controlled Clinical Trial. *Foods* **2020**, *9*, 1449. [CrossRef] [PubMed]

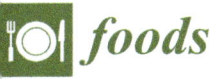

Article

Anti-Apoptotic and Anti-Inflammatory Role of Trans ε-Viniferin in a Neuron–Glia Co-Culture Cellular Model of Parkinson's Disease

Domenico Sergi [1,2], Alex Gélinas [1], Jimmy Beaulieu [1], Justine Renaud [1], Emilie Tardif-Pellerin [1], Jérôme Guillard [3] and Maria-Grazia Martinoli [1,4,*]

[1] Cellular Neurobiology, Department of Medical Biology, Université du Québec, Trois-Rivières, QC G9A 5H7, Canada; Domenico.sergi2@uqtr.ca (D.S.); alex.gelinas2@uqtr.ca (A.G.); jimmyb.92@hotmail.com (J.B.); Justine.renaud@uqtr.ca (J.R.); Emilie.tardif-pellerin@uqtr.ca (E.T.-P.)
[2] Adelaide Medical School, The University of Adelaide, Adelaide, SA 5000, Australia
[3] UMR CNRS 7285 IC2MP, Equipe 5 Synthese Organique, UFR Médecine et Pharmacie, Université de Poitiers, 86073 Poitiers CEDEX 9, France; jerome.guillard@univ-poitiers.fr
[4] Department of Psychiatry and Neuroscience, U. Laval and CHU Research Center, Québec, QC G1V 4G2, Canada
* Correspondence: maria-grazia.martinoli@uqtr.ca

Abstract: The polyphenol trans-ε-viniferin (viniferin) is a dimer of resveratrol, reported to hold antioxidant and anti-inflammatory properties. The aims of our study were to evaluate the neuroprotective potential of viniferin in the nerve growth factor (NGF)-differentiated PC12 cells, a dopaminergic cellular model of Parkinson's disease (PD) and assess its anti-inflammatory properties in a N9 microglia–neuronal PC12 cell co-culture system. The neuronal cells were pre-treated with viniferin, resveratrol or their mixture before the administration of 6-hydroxydopamine (6-OHDA), recognized to induce parkinsonism in rats. Furthermore, N9 microglia cells, in a co-culture system with neuronal PC12, were pre-treated with viniferin, resveratrol or their mixture to investigate whether these polyphenols could reduce lipopolysaccharide (LPS)-induced inflammation. Our results show that viniferin as well as a mixture of viniferin and resveratrol protects neuronal dopaminergic cells from 6-OHDA-induced cytotoxicity and apoptosis. Furthermore, when viniferin, resveratrol or their mixture was used to pre-treat microglia cells in our co-culture system, they reduced neuronal cytotoxicity induced by glial activation. Altogether, our data highlight a novel role for viniferin as a neuroprotective and anti-inflammatory molecule in a dopaminergic cellular model, paving the way for nutraceutical therapeutic avenues in the complementary treatments of PD.

Keywords: trans-ε-viniferin; resveratrol; neuroprotection; oxidative stress; dopamine; apotosis; neuroinflammation; Parkinson's disease

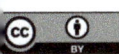

1. Introduction

The incidence of neurodegenerative diseases is increasing worldwide, with Alzheimer's disease (AD) and Parkinson's disease (PD) being the most prevalent. Neurodegenerative diseases are characterized by neuronal loss, which in PD affects the dopaminergic neurons of the substantia nigra pars compacta (SNpc) [1]. Currently, apoptosis triggered by oxidative stress and neuroinflammation appears to be the main driver of dopaminergic neuron loss in PD [2].

Mitochondria are the principal source of reactive oxygen species (ROS), the mandatory bioproducts of oxidative metabolism. Mitochondrial dysfunction, a pivotal pathogenetic feature of PD, exacerbates oxidative stress by fostering ROS production which, in turn, via a feed-forward mechanism worsens mitochondrial dysfunction resulting in the activation of signaling cascades leading to apoptosis [3,4].

Due to their intrinsic low antioxidant activity and to the characteristic dopamine metabolism that generates pro-oxidant byproducts [5], dopaminergic neurons are particularly vulnerable to oxidative stress, which may explain their susceptibility to degeneration typically found in PD.

Besides oxidative stress, neuroinflammation represents another key mechanism responsible for neurodegeneration in PD [6]. In support of this, post mortem investigation in the brain of parkinsonian patients demonstrated elevated levels of activated microglia, and pro-inflammatory cytokines in the substantia nigra and in the striatum [7,8]. However, whether neuroinflammation is a cause or a consequence of neurodegeneration it remains a matter of debate. Nonetheless, in vitro cell co-culture models [9,10], have provided evidence that eliciting a pro-inflammatory phenotype in microglial cells using lipopolysaccharide (LPS), a well know pro-inflammatory molecule, promoted microglia-induced neuronal cell damage [9,11]. To the same extent, stereotaxic LPS injection into the brain of rodents can recapitulate neuroinflammation and promote dopaminergic neuron degeneration [12]. Thus, independently of whether neuroinflammation is involved in the etiology of PD or is the result of nigrostriatal pathway injury, sustained microglia pro-inflammatory activation can contribute to dopaminergic neuron loss.

Nowadays, strategies aimed at tackling oxidative stress and neuroinflammation may represent positive avenues to prevent neurodegeneration. In this regard, bioactive molecules derived from plants have emerged for their neuroprotective potential by countering oxidative stress, inflammation or both. Of these, resveratrol in light of its antioxidant [13] anti-inflammatory [11], and synergistic effects with other polyphenols such as quercetin [11,14,15], is considered one of the most promising. Nonetheless, resveratrol containing foods also present oligomeric forms of stilbenes whose biological effects remain to be fully elucidated, especially with regard to the central nervous system. Of these, ε-viniferin (viniferin), a naturally occurring resveratrol dimer with higher activity and stability, may contribute to the total amount of stilbenes consumed with foods [16]. This molecule shares several health promoting effects with resveratrol, including neuroprotective properties, as demonstrated in animal models of Huntington's disease [17] and AD [18,19]. However, the effect of viniferin on oxidative stress and inflammation-induced injury in dopaminergic neurons remains to be elucidated.

Thus, the aim of this study was to determine whether viniferin was able to prevent 6-hydroxydopamine (6-OHDA)-induced cytotoxicity and apoptosis in a cellular model of PD, PC12 dopaminergic neurons. Furthermore, we aimed at elucidating whether this resveratrol dimer could prevent LPS-activated N9 microglial cells from inducing PC12 cell death in an N9 microglia PC12 cell co-culture system. The effect of viniferin on the aforementioned outcomes was also investigated in the presence of resveratrol, and resveratrol itself was used as reference molecule to benchmark the effect of viniferin. Our results show that viniferin can successfully protect PC12 dopaminergic neurons from oxidative stress-induced apoptosis, and is also able to prevent microglia from promoting neuronal death, with a synergetic effect being observed when resveratrol is used in a mixture together with viniferin.

2. Materials and Methods

2.1. Drugs and Chemicals

All reagents were purchased from Sigma-Aldrich (St. Louis, MO, USA) unless stated otherwise.

2.2. Extractions and Purifications of Polyphenols

Grape canes variety "Ugni" (Vitaceae) were collected from Cognac's vineyards in France. Grape canes were extracted in an extruder (BC21 clextral) apparatus with a mixture of ethanol/water (8/2) as a solvent. The solution was concentrated after filtration, at 40 °C under a vacuum and lyophilized. Dried extract (4 g) was dissolved in 20 mL of a mixture called Biosolvants 1 with the following composition Makigreen D10–EtOAc–EtOH–H_2O, (4:2:3:2) and injected into a centrifugal partition chromatography (CPC) apparatus. The CPC method used to obtain viniferin is the one presented previously [20], but using green solvents as Biosolvent 1 and Biosolvent 2 (Cyclopentane–EtOAc–EtOH–H$_2$O, 1:2:1:2). Thus, fractions were collected and combined on the basis of HPLC analysis, providing a total of three fractions of interest. Fraction 1 (101 mg) corresponded to 95% pure resveratrol as white solid. Fraction 2 (175 mg) contained the dimer of interest, as with viniferin along with other compounds. Afterwards, fraction 2 was re-purified by semi-preparative HPLC and a yellow solid isolated was identified by 1H and 13C NMR spectroscopy analysis in acetone-d6 and mass spectrometry as with viniferin to 98% purity. The concentration of viniferin after extrusion–extraction is very dependent on the grape variety used but with Ugni's grapecane the total polyphenol yield is 0.3% by weight with a concentration of viniferin in the extract grapine-shoot of between 15 and 20%.

2.3. Cell Culture and Treatments

A rat pheochromocytoma cell line (PC12 cells) was obtained from ATCC (Rockville, MD, USA). Cells were maintained in a humidified environment at 37 °C and 5% CO$_2$ atmosphere and routinely grown in RPMI 1640 medium supplemented with 10% heat-inactivated horse serum (HS), 5% heat inactivated fetal bovine serum (FBS; Corning Cellgro, Manassas, VA, USA) and gentamicin (50 µg/mL). Neuronal differentiation was evoked by nerve growth factor-7S (NGF, 50 ng/mL) in RPMI 1640 supplemented with 1% FBS for 9–10 days, as already described [10,21]. NGF-differentiated PC12 cells (neuronal PC12) displayed a dopaminergic phenotype (Figure 1) as already reported [21,22]. They were pretreated with resveratrol or viniferin (generously provided by Dr. Jérôme Guillard, University of Poitiers, Poitiers, France) at 10−9 M or a mixture of the two molecules at 10−9 M for 3 h. Then 6-OHDA (50 µM) or LPS (2 µg/mL) [9] was added to the medium for 24 h. All experiments were performed in RPMI medium without phenol red, supplemented with 1% charcoal-stripped serum to remove steroids from the medium. Microglial cell line N9 was grown in Dulbecco's modified Eagle's medium nutrient mixture F12-Ham's (DMEM-F12) supplemented with 10% HS.

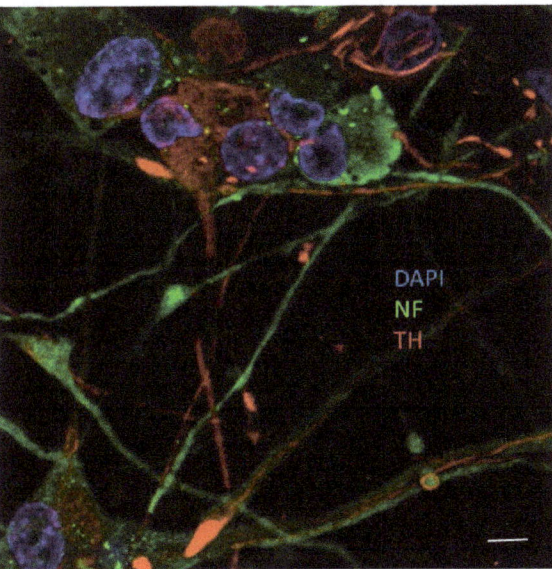

Figure 1. Representative microphotograph of nerve growth factor (NGF)-differentiated PC12 for 9 days by immunofluorescence. Nuclei are counterstained in blue with Dapi. NF: neurofilaments revealed with an anti-neurofilaments antibody (green). TH: tyrosine hydroxylase revealed with an anti-tyrosine antibody as a marker of dopamine (red). Scale bar = 10 µm.

2.4. Neuronal–Glial Co-Culture

Neuronal PC12 cells and N9 microglia were co-cultured without cellular contact to study the impact of LPS-activated microglia on the survival of neuronal cells, as we have already described [9]. In this co-culture system, microglial cells communicate with PC12 neuronal cells through a semipermeable membrane, in the absence of a direct contact between the two cellular systems [23]. Briefly, N9 microglial cells were grown onto culture inserts (pore size 0.4 µm; BD Falcon, Oakville, ON, Canada), LPS (2 µg/mL) was added. After 24 h, inserts containing N9 cells were washed with PBS and then transferred on neuronal PC12, for another 24 h. The PC12 supernatant was collected for cell death measurements with lactate dehydrogenase (LDH) cytotoxicity tests as described below. For immunofluorescent experiment, N9 microglial cells were grown in culture inserts and treated as described then transferred on neuronal PC12 cells grown previously on coverslips [9,11].

2.5. Cytotoxicity Measurements

Cytotoxicity was evaluated using a colorimetric assay based on the quantification of LDH activity released from damaged cells into the cell culture medium, as already described [20]. LDH is a stable cytoplasmic enzyme present in all cells, which is rapidly released into the cell culture supernatant upon plasma membrane damage. Enzyme activity in the cell culture medium is a direct function of lysed cells [24]. Briefly, 100 µL of cell-free culture media served to quantify LDH activity by measuring absorbance at 490 nm using a Thermo Lab Systems (Franklin, MA, USA). Total cellular LDH was determined cells lysed using 1% Triton X-100 (high control); the assay medium was used as a low control and was subtracted from all absorbance measurements:

$$\text{Cytotoxicity (\%)} = (\text{Experimental value-Low control})/(\text{High control-Low control}) \times 100$$

2.6. MTT Assay

The cell metabolic activity was measured using 3-(4,5-dimethyltrazol-2-yl)-2,5-diphenyltetrazolium bromide (MTT) assay [21]. Neuronal PC12 cells, plated in 96-wells plates, were treated as already described and then incubated for 4 h at 37 °C with MTT dye (5 mg/mL), followed by solubilization in SDS 10% and the absorbance was measured at the 595 nm with a microplate reader (Thermo Lab Systems, Franklin, MA, USA).

2.7. Apoptosis- Specific DNA Denaturation Detection

Apoptosis-specific detection of DNA denaturation by formamide was assessed with the single-stranded DNA (ssDNA) apoptosis ELISA kit (Chemicon International, Telok Panglima Garang, Malaysia) as already described [15,22]. This procedure relies the on selective DNA denaturation by formamide in apoptotic cells, which does not occur in necrotic cells nor in cells with DNA damage in the absence of apoptosis [25]. The detection of denatured DNA was performed with a monoclonal antibody highly specific to ssDNA and a peroxidase-labelled secondary antibody on fixed neuronal PC12 cells. Following ssDNA immune detection, the reaction was then terminated with a hydrochloric acid solution and ssDNA was quantified by measuring absorbance at 405 nm in a microplate reader (Thermolab Systems, Vasai-Virar, India). ssDNA was quantified relative to control conditions. Absorbance of positive (wells coated with provided ssDNA) and negative controls (wells coated with S1 nuclease that digest ssDNA) served as quality controls for the ELISA assay, as previously described [26,27].

2.8. Immunofluorescent Microscopy

Apoptotic P12 neuronal cells were detected by both terminal deoxynucleotidyl transferase dUTP nick end labeling (TUNEL, Roche Diagnostics, Basel, Switzerland) and cleaved caspase-3 immunofluorescence. Neuronal PC12 cells were seeded at 25,000 cells/cm^2, differentiated and treated on collagen-coated coverslips in 24-well plates for immunofluorescent microscopy. Briefly, after viniferin and/or resveratrol and/or 6-OHDA treatments, cells were fixed in 4% paraformaldehyde for 15 min at 37 °C, then washed and incubated for 1 h at room temperature in a blocking and permeabilizing solution containing 1% BSA, 0.18% fish skin gelatin, 0.1% Triton X-100 and 0.02% sodium azide [22,26]. Cells were then incubated with anti-cleaved caspase-3 antibody (New England Biolabs, Pickering, ON, Canada) diluted 1:500, for 2 h at room temperature, followed by 90-min incubation with a Cy3-conjugated secondary antibody (Medicorp, Montreal, QC, Canada) diluted 1:500 for 1 h at 4 °C. The coverslips were then transferred to the TUNEL reaction mixture in a humidified atmosphere at 37 °C. The cells were rinsed with PBS, nuclei were counterstained in blue with DAPI for 10 min at 37 °C and mounted with ProLong Antifade kits (Invitrogen). PC12 neuronal cells were considered to be apoptotic when they were positive for cleaved caspase-3 and their nuclei were stained by TUNEL. The number of apoptotic neuronal cells among 300 randomly chosen neuronal cells was counted on 10 different optical fields from 3 slides per group [15], with Pro Express 6.3 software (Media Cybernetics, Rockville, MD, USA).

2.9. Electrophoresis and Immunoblot Analysis

Neuronal cells were grown and treated in 6-well plates. Total proteins were extracted with a Nuclear Extraction Kit (Active Motif, Carlsbad, CA, USA) and their concentration determined by using the BCA protein assay kit (Pierce Biotechnology Inc., Rockford, AZ, USA). Fifteen µg of protein were loaded onto a 12% SDS-polyacrylamide gel. After electrophoretic separation (125 V, for 1 h 30), proteins were transferred onto PVDF membranes (0.22 µm pore size, BioRad) at 25 V overnight. The membranes were blocked in TBST (TBS + Tween 0.05%) with 5% non-fat dry milk for 1 h at room temperature and incubated overnight at 4 °C with primary antibodies: anti-cleaved caspase-3 antibody (1:500) anti-cleaved PARP-1 antibody (1:500) or an anti-β-actin antibody (1:500) (Cell Signaling, Danvers, MA, USA). The blots were then rinsed three times with TBS 0.1% Tween 20 and incubated with peroxidase-conjugated (POD) secondary antibody (1:10,000) for 2 h at room temperature. Blots were washed with TBS 0.1% Tween 20 three times and the signal finally revealed by enhanced chemiluminescence with the AlphaEase FC imaging system (Alpha Innotech, San Leandro, CA, USA) and analyzed with AlphaEase FC software (Alpha Innotech) and ImageJ (imagej.nih.gov).

2.10. ELISA

Pro-inflammatory cytokines IL-1α and TNF-α were measured by specific ELISA kits (BioLegend, San Diego, CA, USA). Following pre-incubation with resveratrol, viniferin, or a mixture of the two molecules for 3 h, N9 microglial cells were administered with LPS 4 µg/mL for 24 h. Supernatants were collected after 27 h and processed for the presence of selected cytokines by ELISA, according to the protocols supplied by the manufacturer. Briefly, the supernatants were collected following the polyphenols and LPS challenges. 96-well plates were coated with mouse-specific monoclonal antibody (IL-1α and TNF-α) and after an overnight incubation, standards and samples were added to the wells for 2 h. The plates were then incubated in the presence of a biotinylated anti-mouse detection antibody for 1 h, followed by a 30 min incubation with an avidin horseradish peroxidase solution. Finally, a tetramethylbenzidine solution was added to the wells for 15 min in the dark to reveal the presence of the cytokines. The reaction was terminated by the addition of 2N sulfuric acid and resulting absorbance recorded at 450 nm using a microplate reader (Synergy H1, BioTek, Winnosky, VT, USA).

2.11. Statistical Analysis

Significant differences between groups were ascertained by One-way analysis of variance (ANOVA), followed by Tukey's post-hoc analysis, performed using the GraphPad Prism8 for Windows (http://www.graphpad.com/). All data were expressed as means ± SEM from at least 3 independent experiments. A p-value < 0.05 was considered statistically significant. Asterisks (*) indicate statistical differences between the treatments and their respective controls (*** $p < 0.001$, ** $p < 0.01$, * $p < 0.05$), plus signs (+) denote statistical differences between the treatments and 6-OHDA (+++ $p < 0.001$, ++ $p < 0.01$, + $p < 0.05$), dollar signs ($) indicate statistical difference between 6-OHDA+resveratrol and 6-OHDA+mixture of the two polyphenols or 6-OHDA and viniferin ($$$ < 0.001, $ < 0.05) and number signs (#) indicates statistical difference between 6-OHDA+viniferin and 6-OHDA + mixture of the two polyphenols (### $p < 0.001$, ## $p < 0.01$). The same symbols were used in the experiments where LPS was used instead of 6-OHDA.

3. Results

3.1. Viniferin Reduced 6-OHDA-Induced Cytotoxicity and Promoted Cell Survival

To evaluate whether viniferin, alone and in combination with resveratrol protected neuronal PC12 cells from 6-OHDA-induced cytotoxicity, we investigated LDH release and metabolic activity in neuronal cells pre-treated for 3 h with resveratrol, viniferin or their combination, before administration of 6-OHDA neurotoxin for 24 h. When the two polyphenols, both at a concentration of 10–9 M, were administered alone before 6-OHDA treatment, they induced a decrease in LDH release by 19 ± 2.5% and 20.3 ± 1.3%, respectively for resveratrol and viniferin (Figure 2A) and increased cellular metabolic activity (Figure 2B) compared to cells treated with 6-OHDA only, by 15.3 ± 0.9% and 14.3 ± 1.9%, respectively. Moreover, preincubation with a mixture of resveratrol and viniferin at a final concentration of 10 -9 M, induced a 27.7 ± 2.3% decrease in LHD release compared to cells exposed to 6-OHDA only (Figure 2A). The same effect was observed for cellular metabolic activity with an increase of 26 ± 2.1% (Figure 2B), notably the effect of the mix of the two polyphenols administered before 6-OHDA challenge was more marked compared to the single polyphenols (Figure 2B).

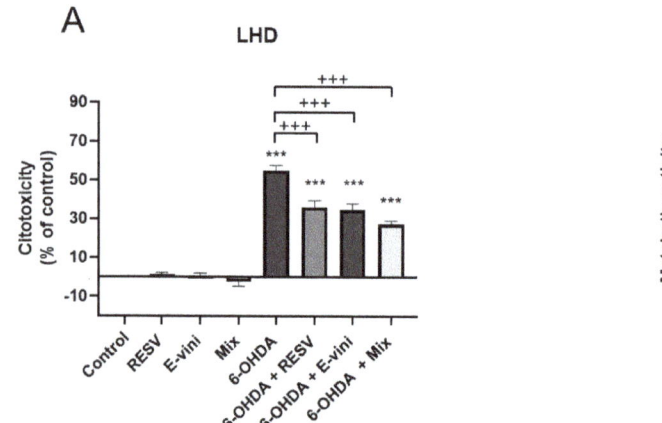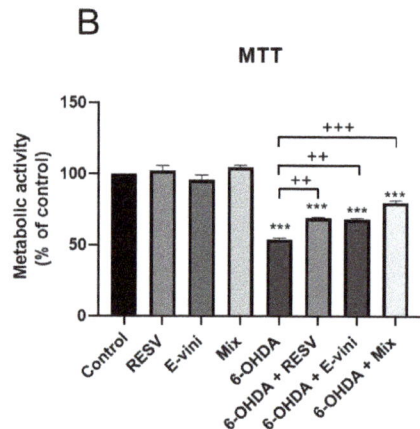

Figure 2. Levels of cytotoxicity (**A**) and metabolic activity (**B**) of PC12 neurons pretreated for three hours with culture medium (control), resveratrol, viniferin or a mixture of both polyphenols (Mix), all at a final concentration of 10–9. Cells were then treated with 6-hydroxydopamine (6-OHDA) at 50 μM for 24 h, as described in the Material and Methods. The supernatants and the cells were used to perform cell death (lactate dehydrogenase (LDH) assay). Data are expressed as means ± SEM of five independent experiments. For each experiment, each condition was in assessed in sextuplicate. Asterisks (*) indicate statistical differences between the treatments and their respective controls (*** $p < 0.001$), plus signs (+) denote statistical differences between 6-OHDA and 6-OHDA in the presence of polyphenols (+++ $p < 0.001$, ++ $p < 0.01$,).

3.2. Viniferin Decreased the Rate of Apoptotic Neuronal PC12 Cells

In order to determine whether polyphenols may counteract cell death by inhibiting the apoptotic cascade, we assessed DNA fragmentation using a ssDNA apoptosis ELISA kit. In line with the results illustrated in Figure 2, resveratrol and viniferin alone or in combination inhibited 6-OHDA-induced DNA fragmentation in neuronal PC12 cells by 52.8 ± 9.6%, 52 ± 9.2% and 55.8 ± 10.3%, respectively (Figure 3A). This result was further confirmed by double immunofluorescence indicating an increase in TUNEL and cleaved caspase-3 positive cells after 6-OHDA treatment (Figure 3B). Notably, this anti-apotoptic effect was more marked when resveratrol and viniferin were used in combination which induced a 36.3 ± 4.2% decrease in the number of apoptotic cells relative to 6-OHDA treated cells, compare to the 22 ± 4% and 25.7 ± 2.3% of resveratrol and viniferin, respectively (Figure 3B).

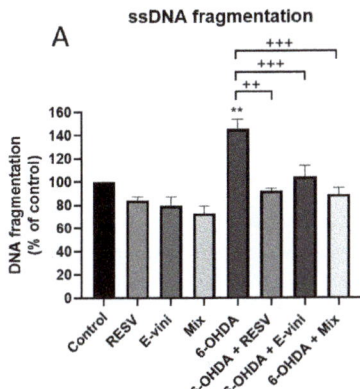 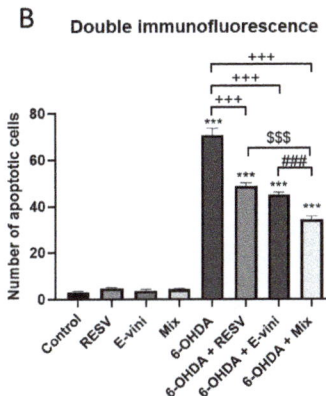

Figure 3. Detection of apoptosis by single stranded (ssDNA) fragmentation (**A**) and by caspase-3 and TUNEL double immunofluorescence (**B**). PC12 neurons pre-treated for three hours with culture medium (control), resveratrol, viniferin or a mixture of both polyphenols (Mix) all at a final concentration of 10^{-9} M. Cells were then treated with 6-OHDA at 50 µM for 24 h, as described in the Material and Methods. Apoptotic neuronal cells among 300 randomly chosen neuronal cells were counted on 10 different optical fields from 3 slides per group, as described in Material and Methods. Data are expressed as means ± SEM of three experiments. For each experiment, each condition was assessed in triplicate. Asterisks (*) indicate statistical differences between the treatments and their respective controls (*** $p < 0.001$, ** $p < 0.01$), plus signs (+) denote statistical differences between 6-OHDA and 6-OHDA in the presence of polyphenols (+++ $p < 0.001$, ++ $p < 0.01$), dollar sign ($) indicates statistical difference between 6-OHDA+resveratrol and 6-OHDA+mixture of the two polyphenols ($$$ < 0.001$) and number sign (#) indicates statistical difference between 6-OHDA+viniferin and 6-OHDA + mixture of the two polyphenols (### $p < 0.001$).

3.3. Viniferin Used Alone or in Combination with Resveratrol Decreased the Cleavage of Caspase-3 and PARP-1 in Neuronal PC12

To further confirm the ability of viniferin to counteract the activation of the apoptotic signaling cascade, we investigated the cleavage of caspase-3 and PARP-1, two dominant markers of early apoptotic signaling, by Western blotting. 6-OHDA increased the cleavage of both caspase-3 and PARP-1 (Figure 4A,B), while these effects were blunted by pre-incubation of neuronal PC12 cells with either viniferin (20.5 ± 0.8% for caspase-3 and 26.1 ± 1.5% forPARP-1), resveratrol (19.8 ± 2.6% for caspase-3 and 27.7 ± 3.3% for PARP-1) or their combination (34.6 ± 2.6 for caspase-3 and 38.9 ± 1.5% for PARP-1) before administration with 6-OHDA (Figure 4A,B). This effect was more pronounced when the mixture of resveratrol and viniferin was administered. In particular, the cleavage of PARP-1 did not increase in the cells pre-treated with the mix of polyphenols compared to control, despite these cells being exposed to 6-OHDA (Figure 4B). These data strongly suggest that, viniferin or resveratrol, used alone or in combination, exerted anti-apoptotic effects, confirming our results illustrated in Figures 2 and 3.

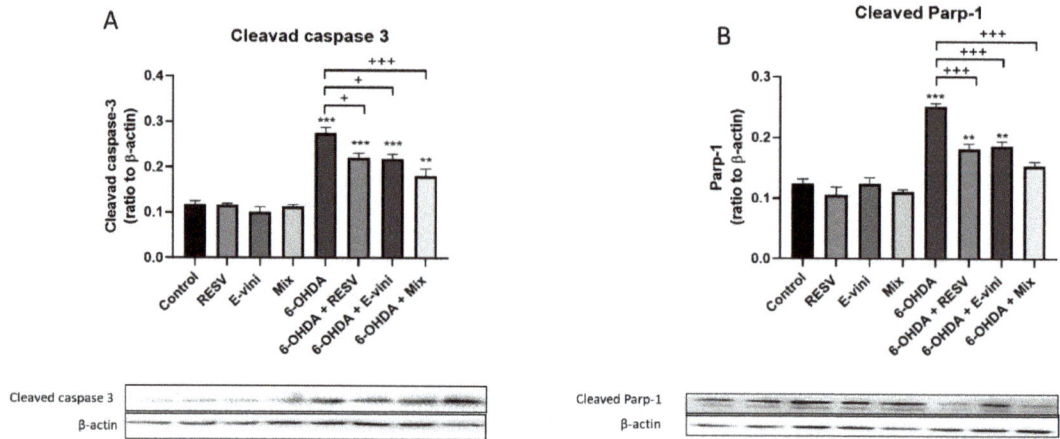

Figure 4. Expression of apoptotic cleaved caspase-3 (**A**) and cleaved Parp-1 (**B**) in PC12 neurons pretreated for three hours with the culture medium (control), resveratrol, viniferin or a mixture of both polyphenols (Mix) at a final concentration of 10−9 M. Cells were then treated with 6-OHDA at 50 µM for 24 h, as described in the Material and Methods. Top panel: Data are expressed as the ratio of cleaved caspase-3 (**A**) or cleaved Parp-1 (**B**) to β-actin. Bottom panel: representative Western blot bands of cleaved caspase-3, cleaved Parp-1 or β-actin. Optical densities were measured on the same membrane. Data are expressed as means ± SEM of three experiments performed in triplicate. Asterisks (*) indicate statistical differences between the treatments and their respective controls (*** $p < 0.001$, ** $p < 0.01$), plus signs (+) denote statistical differences between 6-OHDA and 6-OHDA in the presence of polyphenols (+++ $p < 0.001$, + $p < 0.05$).

3.4. Viniferin, Resveratrol and Their Combination Decreased Neuronal PC12 Cytotoxicity Induced by Activated Microglia, in a Co-Culture System

We have previously demonstrated that LPS-activated N9 microglia cells induced cytotoxicity in neuronal PC12 in a paracrine fashion in a microglia-neuronal PC12 cells co-culture system [9,11]. In order to evaluate whether viniferin may prevent N9 activation and subsequent neuronal PC12 cytotoxicity, N9 cells were pre-treated with the two polyphenols or their mixture and incubated with LPS for 24 h before being co-cultured with PC12 neurons for additional 24 h (Figure 5A). Viniferin, resveratrol and their combination counteracted the increase in LDH release from PC12 neurons co-cultured with LPS-activated N9 microglia, by 51 ± 7.8%, 31.3 ± 5.4% and 64 ± 4.4%, respectively (Figure 5A). This effect was even more marked for viniferin, and the combination of viniferin and resveratrol compared to resveratrol (Figure 5A), suggesting an anti-inflammatory role for viniferin and the mixture of viniferin and resveratrol. Furthermore, to evaluate whether these polyphenols exerted a neuroprotective effect against activated-microglia secretions, neuronal PC12 cells were pretreated with either viniferin, resveratrol or their mixture before being incubated with LPS-stimulated microglial cells (Figure 5B). Viniferin and resveratrol, both alone and in combination, decreased microglia-induced neuronal PC12 cytotoxicity as indicated by a 28.3 ± 2.7%, 21.7 ± 1.5% and 51.3 ± 2% decrease in LDH release, respectively (Figure 5B), suggesting a neuroprotective role for these polyphenols. Notably, the release of LDH was significantly lower for neuronal PC12 pre-treated with the combination of viniferin and resveratrol compared to each independent polyphenol.

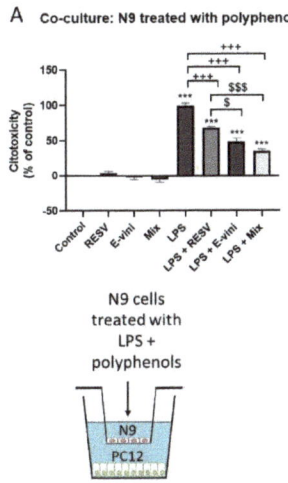
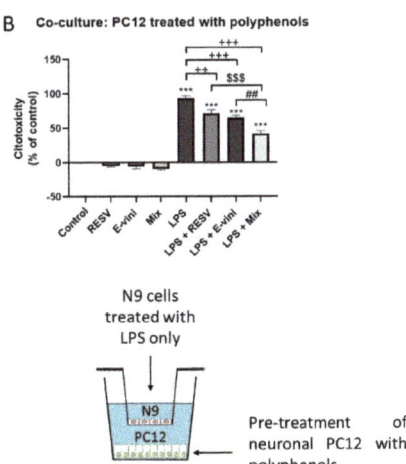

Figure 5. Co-culture of N9 microglial cells on neuronal PC12 cells. (**A**) N9 cells were pre-treated with polyphenols followed incubation with lipopolysaccharide (LPS), as described in the Materials and Methods. (**B**) N9 cells were treated with LPS and neuronal PC12 were pre-incubated with polyphenols as described in the Materials and Methods. Data are expressed as means ± SEM of three experiments. Asterisks (*) indicate statistical differences between the treatments and their respective controls (*** $p < 0.001$), plus signs (+) denote statistical differences between LPS and LPS in the presence of polyphenols. (+++ $p < 0.001$, ++ $p < 0.01$), dollar sign ($) indicates statistical difference between LPS + resveratrol and LPS + mixture of the two polyphenols ($$$ < 0.001, $ < 0.05) and number sign (#) indicates statistical difference between LPS + viniferin and LPS + mixture of the two polyphenols (## $p < 0.01$).

3.5. Viniferin Affected the Secretion of Pro-Inflammatory Cytokines from LPS-Activated N9 Cells

To further investigate the role of viniferin, resveratrol or their mixture on neuroinflammatory mechanisms in N9 microglia-neuronal PC12 cells co-culture, we investigated whether these polyphenols may counteract LPS-induced secretion of pro-inflammatory cytokines. Figure 6 shows that a 24-h LPS treatment increased the secretion of both IL-1α (Figure 6A) and TNFα (Figure 6B). While neither viniferin, resveratrol nor their combination counteracted the secretion of TNFα triggered by LPS (Figure 6B), pre-treating N9 cells with these polyphenols tended to decrease the levels of IL-1α in the cell culture media compared to cells exposed to LPS only (43.3 ± 7.3% for resveratrol; 46.7 ± 11.1% viniferin; 41.5 ± 6.3% for their combination) (Figure 6A).

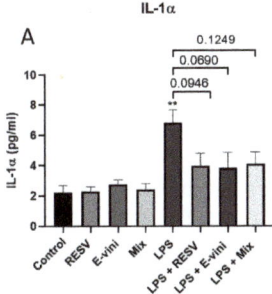
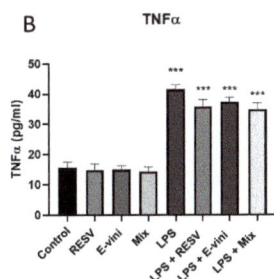

Figure 6. Measurements of cytokine secretion from LPS-activated microglial N9 cells by ELISA specific kit for IL-1α (**A**) and TNFα (**B**). Data are expressed as means ± SEM of four experiments. Asterisks (*) indicate statistical differences between the treatments and their respective controls (*** $p < 0.001$, ** $p < 0.01$).

4. Discussion

This study provides evidence on the neuroprotective and anti-inflammatory potential of the polyphenol viniferin in a cellular model of PD, PC12 dopaminergic neurons, and N9 microglia–PC12 neurons co-culture system [9,10]. These effects were underlie by the ability of this polyphenol to counteract the activation of the apoptotic cascade induced by 6-OHDA in neuronal cells and inhibit cytotoxicity induced by LPS-activated microglia in a microglia–neuron co-culture system. Although our in vitro model could not perfectly replicate in vivo neuron–microglia physiology, these results enlighten that when viniferin was mixed with its homologous resveratrol, it also proved to be more effective in countering neurotoxicity induced by pro-inflammatory activated N9 microglia. Remarkably, despite the fact that final concentration of the mixture of the two polyphenols matched the concentration of the single polyphenols used in isolation, its effect was more powerful in preventing 6-OHDA-induced increase in caspase-3/TUNEL-positive PC12 neurons and inhibiting cytotoxicity promoted by LPS-activated N9 microglia, than resveratrol or viniferin alone.

6-OHDA, due to its similarities to endogenous catecholamines, is taken up and accumulates in catecholaminergic neurons promoting neurotoxicity mainly via oxidative stress-related mechanisms [28]. In support of this, its administration directly into the brain via stereotactic surgery induces parkinsonism in rodent models by promoting nigrostriatal pathway degeneration [29]. These effects were recapitulated in the present study in which 6-OHDA promoted cytotoxicity, as indicated by an increase in LDH release from PC12 dopaminergic neurons and a decrease in their metabolic activity. Importantly, these neurotoxic effects are dependent on the activation of apoptosis as indicated by an increase in caspase-3/TUNEL-positive cells, DNA fragmentation and the cleavage of caspase-3 and PARP, as our present results illustrate.

Nonetheless, despite the deleterious impact of 6-OHDA on cell viability, it was sufficient to administrate the PC12 neuronal cells with resveratrol, viniferin or their combination to inhibit 6-OHDA-induced apoptosis. Of these polyphenols, resveratrol has been widely described for its antioxidant properties [30–33] which are mainly dependent on its ability to induce key transcription factors such as nuclear factor erythroid 2-related factor (Nrf2) and antioxidant enzymes, including glutathione S-transferase (GST) [33,34], all crucial antioxidants defenses [35]. Given the role of oxidative stress in the pathogenesis of neurodegenerative diseases, it represents a promising target to counter neuronal loss [36]. Indeed, resveratrol has been reported to exert neuroprotective effects both in vitro and in vivo [15,37–41], which are in agreement with the results reported herein, most likely dependent on the ability of resveratrol to dampen 6-OHDA-induced oxidative stress triggered by mitochondrial dysfunction [42]. We also investigated in our cell culture system whether a similar effect could be exerted by the naturally occurring resveratrol dimer, viniferin, and if these molecules could act synergically. We report that viniferin was able to inhibit 6-OHDA-induced neurotoxicity and apoptosis to the same extent as resveratrol. These effects, in parallel to those exerted by resveratrol, may be dependent on the antioxidant properties of viniferin [43]. Furthermore, the results reported as part of this study are corroborated by previous evidence supporting the neuroprotective role of viniferin, not only in ADmodels [18,44], but also in PD cellular models [45]. In this regard, in a PD cell model represented by a human neuroblastoma SH-SY5Y cell line exposed to rotenone, viniferin reduced cellular apoptosis, oxidative stress and restored mitochondrial homeostasis, all underlain by SIRT3-mediated fork headbox O3 (FOXO3) deacetylation [45], with FOXO3 playing an important role in PD progression and dopaminergic neuron survival [46]. While this study further supports our results and provide mechanistic insights into the role of viniferin, our data highlight the potency of viniferin considering it was able to inhibit apoptosis at a concentration of 10 nM compared to previous reports using 1 µM for 24 h [45]. Remarkably, the ability of viniferin to counteract apoptosis appeared to be potentiated by resveratrol, with these two molecules acting jointly to increase cellular metabolic activity and decrease the number of caspase-3/TUNEL-positive cells following exposure to 6-OHDA, in our cellular paradigm. Even if the results from cellular paradigms cannot be directly transferred in vivo, we believe that the combination effect of these two molecules represents a promising nutraceutical combination to investigate in in vivo models of PD.

Inflammation represents another pivotal pathogenetic mechanism in PD, underpinned by microglia over-activation which contributes to dopaminergic neuron loss [8,47–49]. In fact, intranigral injection of LPS, a known pro-inflammatory component of Gram-negative bacteria, promotes dopaminergic neuron death recapitulating the pathogenetic features of PD in rodent models [50,51]. This is corroborated with our co-culture model where LPS-activated N9 microglia cells promoted cytotoxicity in downstream neuronal PC12 cells in the absence of a direct cell-to-cell contact, further supporting the role of inflammation in promoting neurotoxicity and its involvement in PD pathogenesis. Furthermore, in consideration of the lack of a direct contact between N9 cells and neurons in our co-culture system, the neurotoxic effect elicited by microglia is mediated by its secretory milieu. Indeed, the activation of the Toll like receptor 4 (TLR4) by LPS in microglial cells triggers the activation of pro-inflammatory pathways, including nuclear factor κB (NFκB) which promotes the secretion of pro-inflammatory cytokines, ROS and nitric oxide via the activation of NADPH oxidase and inducible nitric oxide synthase, respectively [52]. These cytotoxic factors, may also represent the mediators linking microglia activation with PC12 neurons cytotoxicity [53], as indicated in our data by an increase in IL-1α and TNF-α secretion by N9 microglia cells upon exposure to LPS. Remarkably, we demonstrated that resveratrol, viniferin or their combination was able to counteract microglia-induced neurotoxicity both indirectly when these polyphenols were applied to N9 cells, as well as directly when they were used to treat PC12 neurons. This indicates that resveratrol and viniferin were both able to modulate microglia secretory milieu, reducing the cytotoxic effect of microglia secretome by eliciting adaptive protective responses directly in neurons. In either case, resveratrol and viniferin exert anti-inflammatory effects and trigger molecular mechanisms aimed at protecting cells against inflammation and oxidative stress, possibly relying on the activation of the transcription factor nrf2 and the deacetylating enzyme SIRT-3 [17,34]. Particularly, in microglial cells, the activation of nrf2 by resveratrol may be responsible for the inhibition of NFκB via a cross-talk between these transcription factors [54], leading to the consequent downregulation of the inflammatory response elicited by LPS. Similarly, viniferin has also been shown to exert anti-inflammatory responses by inhibition NFκB signaling [55]. Thus, the ability of these polyphenols to restrain activated-microglia from promoting cytotoxicity in PC12 neurons may be dependent on their capacity to dampen LPS-induced inflammation and the consequent release of neurotoxic factors from N9 cells, including nitric oxide, ROS and cytokines. Nonetheless, despite cytokines being a potential driver of microglia-induced neurotoxicity, they are not significantly downregulated by resveratrol or viniferin in our co-culture system. In light of this, these polyphenols may also modulate N9 secretion of neurotoxic mediators such as ROS, nitric oxide and reactive nitrogen species [6,13,52,56,57] that, however, were not measured in our study. Resveratrol and viniferin also exerted direct neuroprotective effect on PC12 neurons co-cultured with activated microglia. This action may rely on the activation of a transcriptional reprogramming triggered by polyphenols in PC12 neurons in order to induce genes involved in cellular defenses, which may be dependent on nrf2 and SIRT-3 activation [17,34]. However, this paradigm remains to be fully elucidated.

To conclude, these polyphenols not only directly protect PC12 neurons against 6-OHDA, but also exert their neuroprotective properties by inhibiting the neurotoxic effect promoted by LPS-activated microglia. Moreover, the neuroprotective potential of resveratrol and viniferin is potentiated when they are used in combination, suggesting a synergistic effect. Thus, considering that the foodstuff rich in resveratrol also contains other forms of stilbenes, including viniferin, and taking into account the neuroprotective potential of their combination, the consumption of these foods may represent a valuable nutritional intervention in complementary therapies for neurodegenerative diseases.

Author Contributions: D.S.: performed the experiments and wrote the manuscript; A.G., J.B. and E.T.-P.: performed the experiments, J.R.: supervised the experiments; J.G.: extracted the polyphenols; M.-G.M. designed, supervised and wrote the manuscript. All authors have read and agreed to the published version of the manuscript.

Funding: This research was funded by NSERC (National Science and Engineering Research Council) of Canada, Discovery grant no. 04321 to M.-G.M.

Data Availability Statement: All data are available upon reasonable request to M.-G. Martinoli.

Acknowledgments: The authors would like to thank Melodie B. Plourde for excellent technical assistance.

Conflicts of Interest: The authors declare no conflict of interest. The funders had no role in the design of the study; in the collection, analyses, or interpretation of data; in the writing of the manuscript, or in the decision to publish the results.

References

1. Hornykiewicz, O. The discovery of dopamine deficiency in the parkinsonian brain. *J. Neural Transm. Suppl.* **2006**, 9–15. [CrossRef]
2. Tatton, W.G.; Chalmers-Redman, R.; Brown, D.; Tatton, N. Apoptosis in Parkinson's disease: Signals for neuronal degradation. *Ann. Neurol.* **2003**, *53* (Suppl. 3), S61–S70. [CrossRef]
3. Fiskum, G.; Starkov, A.; Polster, B.M.; Chinopoulos, C. Mitochondrial mechanisms of neural cell death and neuroprotective interventions in Parkinson's disease. *Ann. N. Y. Acad. Sci.* **2003**, *991*, 111–119. [CrossRef] [PubMed]
4. Sergi, D.; Renaud, J.; Simola, N.; Martinoli, M.G. Diabetes, a Contemporary Risk for Parkinson's Disease: Epidemiological and Cellular Evidences. *Front. Aging Neurosci.* **2019**, *11*, 302. [CrossRef]
5. Cohen, G. Oxy-radical toxicity in catecholamine neurons. *Neurotoxicology* **1984**, *5*, 77–82. [PubMed]
6. Tansey, M.G.; Goldberg, M.S. Neuroinflammation in Parkinson's disease: Its role in neuronal death and implications for therapeutic intervention. *Neurobiol. Dis.* **2010**, *37*, 510–518. [CrossRef]
7. McGeer, P.L.; Itagaki, S.; Boyes, B.E.; McGeer, E.G. Reactive microglia are positive for HLA-DR in the substantia nigra of Parkinson's and Alzheimer's disease brains. *Neurology* **1988**, *38*, 1285–1291. [CrossRef]
8. Gelders, G.; Baekelandt, V.; Van der P56erren, A. Linking Neuroinflammation and Neurodegeneration in Parkinson's Disease. *J. Immunol. Res.* **2018**, *2018*, 4784268. [CrossRef]
9. Renaud, J.; Martinoli, M.G. Development of an Insert Co-culture System of Two Cellular Types in the Absence of Cell-Cell Contact. *J. Vis. Exp.* **2016**, e54356. [CrossRef]
10. Bournival, J.; Plouffe, M.; Renaud, J.; Provencher, C.; Martinoli, M.G. Quercetin and sesamin protect dopaminergic cells from MPP+-induced neuroinflammation in a microglial (N9)-neuronal (PC12) coculture system. *Oxid. Med. Cell. Longev.* **2012**, *2012*, 921941. [CrossRef] [PubMed]
11. Bureau, G.; Longpre, F.; Martinoli, M.G. Resveratrol and quercetin, two natural polyphenols, reduce apoptotic neuronal cell death induced by neuroinflammation. *J. Neurosci. Res.* **2008**, *86*, 403–410. [CrossRef]
12. Liu, M.; Bing, G. Lipopolysaccharide animal models for Parkinson's disease. *Parkinsons Dis.* **2011**, *2011*, 327089. [CrossRef]
13. Aquilano, K.; Baldelli, S.; Rotilio, G.; Ciriolo, M.R. Role of nitric oxide synthases in Parkinson's disease: A review on the antioxidant and anti-inflammatory activity of polyphenols. *Neurochem. Res.* **2008**, *33*, 2416–2426. [CrossRef]
14. Zamin, L.L.; Filippi-Chiela, E.C.; Dillenburg-Pilla, P.; Horn, F.; Salbego, C.; Lenz, G. Resveratrol and quercetin cooperate to induce senescence-like growth arrest in C6 rat glioma cells. *Cancer Sci.* **2009**, *100*, 1655–1662. [CrossRef]
15. Bournival, J.; Quessy, P.; Martinoli, M.G. Protective effects of resveratrol and quercetin against MPP+-induced oxidative stress act by modulating markers of apoptotic death in dopaminergic neurons. *Cell. Mol. Neurobiol.* **2009**, *29*, 1169–1180. [CrossRef] [PubMed]
16. El Khawand, T.; Courtois, A.; Valls, J.; Richard, T.; Krisa, S. A review of dietary stilbenes: Sources and bioavailability. *Phytochem. Rev.* **2018**, *17*, 1007–1029. [CrossRef]
17. Fu, J.; Jin, J.; Cichewicz, R.H.; Hageman, S.A.; Ellis, T.K.; Xiang, L.; Peng, Q.; Jiang, M.; Arbez, N.; Hotaling, K.; et al. trans-(-)-epsilon-Viniferin increases mitochondrial sirtuin 3 (SIRT3), activates AMP-activated protein kinase (AMPK), and protects cells in models of Huntington Disease. *J. Biol. Chem.* **2012**, *287*, 24460–24472. [CrossRef] [PubMed]
18. Caillaud, M.; Guillard, J.; Richard, D.; Milin, S.; Chassaing, D.; Paccalin, M.; Page, G.; Rioux Bilan, A. Trans epsilon viniferin decreases amyloid deposits and inflammation in a mouse transgenic Alzheimer model. *PLoS ONE* **2019**, *14*, e0212663. [CrossRef]
19. Vion, E.; Page, G.; Bourdeaud, E.; Paccalin, M.; Guillard, J.; Rioux Bilan, A. Trans epsilon-viniferin is an amyloid-beta disaggregating and anti-inflammatory drug in a mouse primary cellular model of Alzheimer's disease. *Mol. Cell. Neurosci.* **2018**, *88*, 1–6. [CrossRef]
20. Houille, B.; Papon, N.; Boudesocque, L.; Bourdeaud, E.; Besseau, S.; Courdavault, V.; Enguehard-Gueiffier, C.; Delanoue, G.; Guerin, L.; Bouchara, J.P.; et al. Antifungal activity of resveratrol derivatives against Candida species. *J. Nat. Prod.* **2014**, *77*, 1658–1662. [CrossRef]

21. Gelinas, S.; Martinoli, M.G. Neuroprotective effect of estradiol and phytoestrogens on MPP+-induced cytotoxicity in neuronal PC12 cells. *J. Neurosci. Res.* **2002**, *70*, 90–96. [CrossRef] [PubMed]
22. Arel-Dubeau, A.M.; Longpre, F.; Bournival, J.; Tremblay, C.; Demers-Lamarche, J.; Haskova, P.; Attard, E.; Germain, M.; Martinoli, M.G. Cucurbitacin E has neuroprotective properties and autophagic modulating activities on dopaminergic neurons. *Oxid. Med. Cell. Longev.* **2014**, *2014*, 425496. [CrossRef] [PubMed]
23. Li, F.Q.; Wang, T.; Pei, Z.; Liu, B.; Hong, J.S. Inhibition of microglial activation by the herbal flavonoid baicalein attenuates inflammation-mediated degeneration of dopaminergic neurons. *J. Neural Transm.* **2005**, *112*, 331–347. [CrossRef] [PubMed]
24. Decker, T.; Lohmann-Matthes, M.L. A quick and simple method for the quantitation of lactate dehydrogenase release in measurements of cellular cytotoxicity and tumor necrosis factor (TNF) activity. *J. Immunol. Methods* **1988**, *115*, 61–69. [CrossRef]
25. Frankfurt, O.S.; Krishan, A. Identification of apoptotic cells by formamide-induced dna denaturation in condensed chromatin. *J. Histochem. Cytochem.* **2001**, *49*, 369–378. [CrossRef]
26. Renaud, J.; Bournival, J.; Zottig, X.; Martinoli, M.G. Resveratrol protects DAergic PC12 cells from high glucose-induced oxidative stress and apoptosis: Effect on p53 and GRP75 localization. *Neurotox. Res.* **2014**, *25*, 110–123. [CrossRef]
27. Carange, J.; Longpre, F.; Daoust, B.; Martinoli, M.G. 24-Epibrassinolide, a Phytosterol from the Brassinosteroid Family, Protects Dopaminergic Cells against MPP-Induced Oxidative Stress and Apoptosis. *J. Toxicol.* **2011**, *2011*, 392859. [CrossRef]
28. Simola, N.; Morelli, M.; Carta, A.R. The 6-hydroxydopamine model of Parkinson's disease. *Neurotox. Res.* **2007**, *11*, 151–167. [CrossRef] [PubMed]
29. Quiroga-Varela, A.; Aguilar, E.; Iglesias, E.; Obeso, J.A.; Marin, C. Short- and long-term effects induced by repeated 6-OHDA intraventricular administration: A new progressive and bilateral rodent model of Parkinson's disease. *Neuroscience* **2017**, *361*, 144–156. [CrossRef]
30. Kim, D.W.; Kim, Y.M.; Kang, S.D.; Han, Y.M.; Pae, H.O. Effects of Resveratrol and trans-3,5,4'-Trimethoxystilbene on Glutamate-Induced Cytotoxicity, Heme Oxygenase-1, and Sirtuin 1 in HT22 Neuronal Cells. *Biomol. Ther.* **2012**, *20*, 306–312. [CrossRef]
31. Son, Y.; Byun, S.J.; Pae, H.O. Involvement of heme oxygenase-1 expression in neuroprotection by piceatannol, a natural analog and a metabolite of resveratrol, against glutamate-mediated oxidative injury in HT22 neuronal cells. *Amino Acids* **2013**, *45*, 393–401. [CrossRef] [PubMed]
32. Truong, V.L.; Jun, M.; Jeong, W.S. Role of resveratrol in regulation of cellular defense systems against oxidative stress. *Biofactors* **2018**, *44*, 36–49. [CrossRef]
33. Arbo, B.D.; Andre-Miral, C.; Nasre-Nasser, R.G.; Schimith, L.E.; Santos, M.G.; Costa-Silva, D.; Muccillo-Baisch, A.L.; Hort, M.A. Resveratrol Derivatives as Potential Treatments for Alzheimer's and Parkinson's Disease. *Front. Aging Neurosci.* **2020**, *12*, 103. [CrossRef] [PubMed]
34. Farkhondeh, T.; Folgado, S.L.; Pourbagher-Shahri, A.M.; Ashrafizadeh, M.; Samarghandian, S. The therapeutic effect of resveratrol: Focusing on the Nrf2 signaling pathway. *Biomed. Pharm.* **2020**, *127*, 110234. [CrossRef] [PubMed]
35. Munialo, C.D.; Naumovski, N.; Sergi, D.; Stewart, D.; Mellor, D.D. Critical evaluation of the extrapolation of data relative to antioxidant function from the laboratory and their implications on food production and human health: A review. *Int. J. Food Sci. Technol.* **2019**. [CrossRef]
36. Blesa, J.; Trigo-Damas, I.; Quiroga-Varela, A.; Jackson-Lewis, V.R. Oxidative stress and Parkinson's disease. *Front. Neuroanat* **2015**, *9*, 91. [CrossRef]
37. Zhang, J.; Fan, W.; Wang, H.; Bao, L.; Li, G.; Li, T.; Song, S.; Li, H.; Hao, J.; Sun, J. Resveratrol Protects PC12 Cell against 6-OHDA Damage via CXCR4 Signaling Pathway. *Evid. Based Complement. Altern. Med.* **2015**, *2015*, 730121. [CrossRef]
38. Wang, H.; Dong, X.; Liu, Z.; Zhu, S.; Liu, H.; Fan, W.; Hu, Y.; Hu, T.; Yu, Y.; Li, Y.; et al. Resveratrol Suppresses Rotenone-induced Neurotoxicity Through Activation of SIRT1/Akt1 Signaling Pathway. *Anat. Rec.* **2018**, *301*, 1115–1125. [CrossRef]
39. Huang, N.; Zhang, Y.; Chen, M.; Jin, H.; Nie, J.; Luo, Y.; Zhou, S.; Shi, J.; Jin, F. Resveratrol delays 6-hydroxydopamine-induced apoptosis by activating the PI3K/Akt signaling pathway. *Exp. Gerontol.* **2019**, *124*, 110653. [CrossRef]
40. Palle, S.; Neerati, P. Improved neuroprotective effect of resveratrol nanoparticles as evinced by abrogation of rotenone-induced behavioral deficits and oxidative and mitochondrial dysfunctions in rat model of Parkinson's disease. *Naunyn Schmiedebergs Arch. Pharm.* **2018**, *391*, 445–453. [CrossRef]
41. Blanchet, J.; Longpre, F.; Bureau, G.; Morissette, M.; DiPaolo, T.; Bronchti, G.; Martinoli, M.G. Resveratrol, a red wine polyphenol, protects dopaminergic neurons in MPTP-treated mice. *Prog. Neuropsychopharmacol. Biol. Psychiatry* **2008**, *32*, 1243–1250. [CrossRef]
42. Kupsch, A.; Schmidt, W.; Gizatullina, Z.; Debska-Vielhaber, G.; Voges, J.; Striggow, F.; Panther, P.; Schwegler, H.; Heinze, H.J.; Vielhaber, S.; et al. 6-Hydroxydopamine impairs mitochondrial function in the rat model of Parkinson's disease: Respirometric, histological, and behavioral analyses. *J. Neural Transm.* **2014**, *121*, 1245–1257. [CrossRef]
43. Kong, Q.; Ren, X.; Hu, R.; Yin, X.; Jiang, G.; Pan, Y. Isolation and purification of two antioxidant isomers of resveratrol dimer from the wine grape by counter-current chromatography. *J. Sep. Sci.* **2016**, *39*, 2374–2379. [CrossRef]
44. Jeong, H.Y.; Kim, J.Y.; Lee, H.K.; Ha, D.T.; Song, K.S.; Bae, K.; Seong, Y.H. Leaf and stem of Vitis amurensis and its active components protect against amyloid beta protein (25–35)-induced neurotoxicity. *Arch. Pharm. Res.* **2010**, *33*, 1655–1664. [CrossRef]
45. Zhang, S.; Ma, Y.; Feng, J. Neuroprotective mechanisms of epsilon-viniferin in a rotenone-induced cell model of Parkinson's disease: Significance of SIRT3-mediated FOXO3 deacetylation. *Neural Regen. Res.* **2020**, *15*, 2143–2153. [CrossRef] [PubMed]

46. Pino, E.; Amamoto, R.; Zheng, L.; Cacquevel, M.; Sarria, J.C.; Knott, G.W.; Schneider, B.L. FOXO3 determines the accumulation of alpha-synuclein and controls the fate of dopaminergic neurons in the substantia nigra. *Hum. Mol. Genet.* **2014**, *23*, 1435–1452. [CrossRef] [PubMed]
47. Gyoneva, S.; Shapiro, L.; Lazo, C.; Garnier-Amblard, E.; Smith, Y.; Miller, G.W.; Traynelis, S.F. Adenosine A2A receptor antagonism reverses inflammation-induced impairment of microglial process extension in a model of Parkinson's disease. *Neurobiol. Dis.* **2014**, *67*, 191–202. [CrossRef] [PubMed]
48. Deleidi, M.; Gasser, T. The role of inflammation in sporadic and familial Parkinson's disease. *Cell. Mol. Life Sci.* **2013**, *70*, 4259–4273. [CrossRef] [PubMed]
49. McGeer, P.L.; McGeer, E.G. Inflammation and neurodegeneration in Parkinson's disease. *Parkinsonism Relat. Disord.* **2004**, *10* (Suppl. 1), S3–S7. [CrossRef]
50. Castano, A.; Herrera, A.J.; Cano, J.; Machado, A. Lipopolysaccharide intranigral injection induces inflammatory reaction and damage in nigrostriatal dopaminergic system. *J. Neurochem.* **1998**, *70*, 1584–1592. [CrossRef]
51. Herrera, A.J.; Castano, A.; Venero, J.L.; Cano, J.; Machado, A. The single intranigral injection of LPS as a new model for studying the selective effects of inflammatory reactions on dopaminergic system. *Neurobiol. Dis.* **2000**, *7*, 429–447. [CrossRef] [PubMed]
52. Zhao, J.; Bi, W.; Xiao, S.; Lan, X.; Cheng, X.; Zhang, J.; Lu, D.; Wei, W.; Wang, Y.; Li, H.; et al. Neuroinflammation induced by lipopolysaccharide causes cognitive impairment in mice. *Sci. Rep.* **2019**, *9*, 5790. [CrossRef] [PubMed]
53. Simpson, D.S.A.; Oliver, P.L. ROS Generation in Microglia: Understanding Oxidative Stress and Inflammation in Neurodegenerative Disease. *Antioxidants* **2020**, 743. [CrossRef] [PubMed]
54. Wardyn, J.D.; Ponsford, A.H.; Sanderson, C.M. Dissecting molecular cross-talk between Nrf2 and NF-kappaB response pathways. *Biochem. Soc. Trans.* **2015**, *43*, 621–626. [CrossRef] [PubMed]
55. Ha, D.T.; Long, P.T.; Hien, T.T.; Tuan, D.T.; An, N.T.T.; Khoi, N.M.; Van Oanh, H.; Hung, T.M. Anti-inflammatory effect of oligostilbenoids from Vitis heyneana in LPS-stimulated RAW 264.7 macrophages via suppressing the NF-kappaB activation. *Chem. Cent. J.* **2018**, *12*, 14. [CrossRef]
56. Fischer, R.; Maier, O. Interrelation of oxidative stress and inflammation in neurodegenerative disease: Role of TNF. *Oxid. Med. Cell. Longev.* **2015**, *2015*, 610813. [CrossRef] [PubMed]
57. Bournival, J.; Francoeur, M.A.; Renaud, J.; Martinoli, M.G. Quercetin and sesamin protect neuronal PC12 cells from high-glucose-induced oxidation, nitrosative stress, and apoptosis. *Rejuvenation Res.* **2012**, *15*, 322–333. [CrossRef]

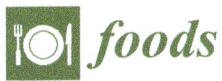

Article

Effect of a Nutritional Support System (Diet and Supplements) for Improving Gross Motor Function in Cerebral Palsy: An Exploratory Randomized Controlled Clinical Trial

Fernando Leal-Martínez [1], Denise Franco [1], Andrea Peña-Ruiz [1], Fabiola Castro-Silva [2], Andrea A. Escudero-Espinosa [2], Oscar G. Rolón-Lacarrier [3], Mardia López-Alarcón [4], Ximena De León [1], Mariana Linares-Eslava [1] and Antonio Ibarra [1,*]

1. Centro de Investigación en Ciencias de la Salud (CICSA), FCS, Universidad Anáhuac México Norte, Huixquilucan 52786, Mexico; ferman5@hotmail.com (F.L.-M.); iantonio65@yahoo.com (D.F.); iantonio65@gmail.com (A.P.-R.); ceciggg73@gmail.com (X.D.L.); liesmari@hotmail.com (M.L.-E.)
2. Departamento de Terapia Física, Centro de Rehabilitación e Inclusión Infantil Teletón (CRIT), Tlalnepantla de Baz 54010, Mexico; juan.ibarra@softhealth.com.mx (F.C.-S.); andyibarra03@gmail.com (A.A.E.-E.)
3. Departamento de Investigación y Enseñanza, Centro de Rehabilitación e Inclusión Infantil Teletón (CRIT), Tlalnepantla de Baz 54010, Mexico; edyibarra05@gmail.com
4. Unidad de Investigación Médica en Nutrición, Hospital de Pediatría CMN siglo XXI, Ciudad de Mexico 06720, Mexico; mardyalo@hotmail.com
* Correspondence: jose.ibarra@anahuac.mx; Tel.: +52-5554-197-603

Received: 27 July 2020; Accepted: 1 October 2020; Published: 13 October 2020

Abstract: Background: Most patients with cerebral palsy (CP) do not respond to physical therapy due to deterioration in their nutritional status, secondary to gastrointestinal disorders and the catabolic state of the disease itself. However, basic treatments only contemplate the energy requirements and do not consider supplementation with glutamine, zinc, selenium, colecalciferol, spirulina, omega 3 or even vegetal proteins. Objective: In this study, we determined the effect of using a nutritional support system (NSS): diet and supplements, on the gross motor function in children with CP with spastic diparesic and Gross Motor Function Classification System III (GMFCS III). Methods: An exploratory study was performed. Thirty patients (from 4 to 12 years old) were randomly assigned to: (1) dietary surveillance (FG), (2) deworming and WHO diet (CG), or (3) deworming and the NSS (IG). Gross motor function was evaluated using the gross motor function measure (GMFM) scale. Results: The IG-treated group presented a significant improvement in standing and walking parameters analyzed in the GMFM compared with FG and CG groups. Fifty percent of the IG-treated patients managed to walk, while in the other groups, no patients were able to walk. Conclusions: The NSS used in the present work improves gross motor function and promotes walking in patients with CP.

Keywords: child; cerebral palsy; diet modification; motor development delay; nutrition disorder; nutritional support

1. Introduction

Cerebral palsy (CP) is the most common physical disability in childhood. Its prevalence worldwide and in developed countries is approximated to 2–2.5 cases per 1000 live births [1,2]. According to the Center for Disease Control (CDC), the cost per person of CP was estimated at around 921,000 dollars per year in the United States (2003), while the costs for general medical assistance amounted to

11,500 million dollars [3]. CP is a permanent movement disorder characterized by a persistent postural tone, causing limitation of activity. This is attributed to non-progressive damage on a developing and immature brain that is originated in the fetal, perinatal period (greater percentage), or first years of life. CP is accompanied by alterations in sensation, cognition, communication, perception, spasticity, seizures, disorders in swallowing, and malnutrition [4].

Traditional treatment for patients with CP generates a recovery of 2% [5] per year and is based on rehabilitation, botulinum toxin therapy, general care, and in the case of malnutrition or disorders in swallowing, nutritional support which is based on the adaptation of Krick to the Schofield formula [5,6]. Nevertheless, there are no specific recommendations for dietary intake in patients with CP. Moreover, the literature information about nutritional support for improving neurological function is scarce. That is why CP continues to be the focus of numerous investigations. In line with this, a novel strategy that includes nutrition and neurological remodeling support could be of valuable use for patients with CP since, at the same time that it nourishes, it significantly impacts the neurological recovery of the patient, especially motor function. Gross motor dysfunction is one of the main affectations in children with CP [7], and it is associated with spasticity, which reflects the damage in the Pyramidal System. This movement-alteration is also strongly associated with malnutrition in patients with CP [8]. Currently, the use of functional foods, supplements or even the administration of probiotics or prebiotics as a therapeutic strategy has become a very important research area [9]. In this field, numerous studies have tested—separately—the effect of some nutrients in the central nervous system (CNS); however, there are no investigations integrating these elements as a whole treatment in CP. Arginine, for instance, participates in the formation of nitric oxide (NO) which is associated with neuronal regeneration and protection of the CNS [10]. Docosahexaenoic acid (DHA) and sphingosine 1 phosphate (S1P) prevent the early death of newly generated neurons [11]. Omega 3 polyunsaturated fatty acids (PUFAs n-3) participate in brain plasticity, neurogenesis, and memory and brain repair. Neuromuscular alterations after cerebral ischemia, improve after omega-3 treatment [12,13]. On the other hand, supplementation with probiotics has also been proposed as a therapeutic strategy for alleviating CNS pathologies [14]. Probiotics have been used to stimulate the production of neurotransmitters, memory, neuroregeneration, and also for correcting malabsorption [15]. In this work, probiotics were used for the latter purpose.

In order to provide patients with CP with the best therapeutic strategy, it is also important to consider the use of several metabolic rescue pathways to produce energy, including lactate and alanine cycles, where glutamine and glutamic acid are the main substrates [16]. Deficiencies in plasma concentrations of iron, folate, niacin, calcium, vitamins D and E, zinc, selenium, and proteins have been in reported in children with CP, even in children who were being supplemented. Therefore, supplementation of some nutrients and proteins should also be considered [17–19]. Regarding protein supplementation, it is relevant to mention that protein plant supplements such as Spirulina Maxima, in addition to providing a high protein intake, produce compounds such as PUFAs and are also a good source of vitamins [20].

Finally, it is relevant to consider that 3500 million people in the world are parasitized and of them, the majority are children [21]. This, and other factors such as the catabolic increment observed in neurologic patients, difficulties for feeding mechanics, gastrointestinal alterations, and the use of drugs that compete with the transport, absorption, or metabolism of nutrients, increases the risk of malnutrition in children with CP [22,23]. Therefore, parasitosis makes malnutrition an even more significant problem in this group of people.

It can be said, therefore, that there are several factors that need to be addressed in order to establish the best therapeutic strategy for CP. At the moment, there is no scientific evidence of an integrative nutritional support. That is why, in the present study, we tested an integral food system—the nutritional support system (NSS)—that includes nutrition, metabolic support, deworming, and neurological remodeling support.

2. Materials and Methods

The exploratory study was designed as a controlled clinical trial which was randomized, and blinded; children with CP with spastic diparesis and GMFCS III were enrolled in this study (during a period of 3 years) and treated at the Children's Telethon Rehabilitation Center (CRIT) in Tlalnepantla Estado de México. The duration of the study was 13 weeks for each participant.

The trial complied with the principles of the Declaration of Helsinki and the Mexican norm NOM-012-SSA3-2012 for scientific research in humans. All procedures were approved by the Committee of Research of the Faculty of Health Sciences of the Universidad Anáhuac México Campus Norte with the number 2014/03001. The parent or guardian and the patient (in the event that they could sign) signed the informed consent letter voluntarily. The Clinical Trials identifier of this study is: NCT03933709.

2.1. Participants

Fifty-three children were interviewed and, from this group, thirty met the inclusion criteria (see Figure 1).

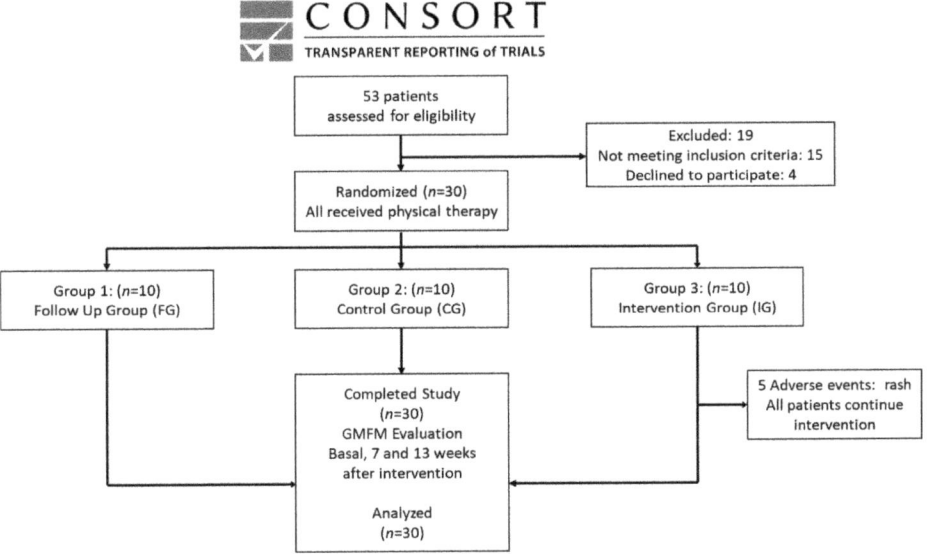

Figure 1. Consort, transparent reporting of trials.

Inclusion criteria: Patients with CP with spastic diparesis and GMFCS III (these patients demonstrate elevated functionality in the categories of lying/rolling, sitting, and crawling), of both genders aged between 4 and 12 years old, who had support from a full-time caregiver, and who were able to feed orally.

Non-inclusion criteria: Patients with CP presenting another catabolic disease which could increase the risk of malnutrition (renal, cardiovascular, pulmonary, hepatic, or immunological disease), and those presenting infections or receiving antibiotic treatment at least 15 days before starting the study; patients who had received therapy with botulinum toxin or muscle relaxants in the last 6 months; patients with CP presenting severe gastroesophageal reflux or with any type of surgery performed in the last 9 months; and patients walking by themselves.

2.2. Group Assignments

Before recruiting patients, thirty numbers (from 1 to 30) were placed in a tombola. Afterwards, each number was randomly selected from the tombola and sequentially allocated to one of three groups, until reaching 10 numbers per group. Each number represented the time the patient was to be enrolled. This way, once initiated the recruitment, the first patient was assigned number one; the second was number two, and so on. In this fashion, each patient was allocated (according to the time of enrollment) to the group to which, their number corresponded.

Afterwards, the patients were informed and trained according to their corresponding groups: (1) the Follow-up Group (FG, $n = 10$)—only their usual diet was monitored; (2) the Control Group (CG, $n = 10$) was dewormed and received the nutritional therapy recommended by the WHO [23]; (3) the Intervention Group (IG, $n = 10$) was dewormed and received the NSS. As parasitosis is a common variable that could affect the absorption of nutrients among the groups and, as a part of our hypothesis, is related to the positive effect that deworming could have on the absorption of supplements, we decided to contrast the IG group versus a dewormed (CG) group and a non-dewormed (FG) group.

All participants received Bobath physical therapy.

2.3. Procedures

Once the participants were selected, parents and children with CP were called to explain the protocol and to collect their informed consent forms. Upon entering the study, the nutritional history and gross motor function measure (GMFM) scale qualification was obtained and recorded from each patient. Thereafter, patients with CP were randomly allocated into the 3 groups (FG, CG, and IG). The energy calculation for the CG and IG groups was performed with the Krick formula (50% carbohydrates, 30% lipids, and 20% proteins).

The parents and/or caregivers of the participants were trained on the project, procedures, as well as feeding and supplementation schemes if required. They were also warned to avoid any comment on the treatment that the patient received. At the beginning of the treatment, the CG and IG groups were dewormed with nitazoxanide at a dosage of 7.5 mg/kg every 12 h for 3 days.

2.4. Diet, Shakes, and Supplementation

Our nutritional support system consists of a shake-based diet with functional ingredients, high levels of vegetables, fruits, cereals, root-vegetables, and fish. Additionally, it is supplemented with glutamine, arginine, folic acid, nicotinic acid, zinc, selenium, cholecalciferol, ascorbic acid, spirulina, vegetal protein, PUFAs n-3, and probiotics (Saccharomyces Boulardii; 200 mg every 12 h for 3 days in the basal period and at week 7, for correcting malabsorption). In order to ensure that patients reached the necessary caloric intake, they were instructed to take two shakes in the morning and one in the evening. Shakes were made at home by the parents and consumed immediately after preparation. A shake-based diet was chosen since it facilitates nutrient absorption in the intestine. Envelopes containing the ingredients for the shakes were provided to encourage consumption of the shakes and to make it easier to adhere to the therapy. The IG supplements were mixed in numbered envelopes and administered in three shakes: Shakes 1 and 3 contained amaranth ($1\frac{1}{2}$ tablespoon), oats ($1\frac{1}{2}$ tablespoon), 1/4 of a medium avocado, 1 medium-sized banana, egg whites (two), cinnamon (1 g) and almond milk (250 mL)—equivalent to 650 kcal, 14 g of protein, 11 g of lipids, and 58 g of carbohydrates. Shake 2 contained celery (1/2 of the stalk), oranges (two), pineapple (100 g), nopal (1/2 of a medium leaf), 1 sprig of parsley, radish (1/4 of a medium radish), and ginger (3 g) equivalent to 148 kcal, 3.5 g of protein, 3.5 g of lipids, and 36 g of carbohydrates and was to be drunk in the morning together with shake 1 (see Figure 2).The ingredients and administration of the envelopes were as follows: Envelope 1 contained 4.9 g of Spirulina Maxima, 100 mg ascorbic acid, 5 mg folic acid, and 10 g of glutamine. This envelope was to be added to shake 1 during the first 10 days of the intervention. Envelope 2 contained 1g PUFAs n-3 and was to be added to shake 2 which was given throughout the intervention. Envelope 3 contained 4.9 g of Spirulina Maxima, 100 mg ascorbic acid, 5 mg folic acid, 5.2 g vegetable protein, 125 mg nicotinic acid, 50 mg zinc, 100 mcg selenium and 800 UI cholecalciferol. This envelope was to be added to shake 1 from day 11 until the end of week 6, after which it was suspended for 10 days and substituted for envelope 5 and then to be retaken until the end of the intervention. Envelope 4 contained 1 g arginine and was to be added to shake 3 from day 8 until the end of the intervention. Envelope 5 contained the same ingredients as envelope 3 with an additional 10 g glutamine and was to be added to shake 1 from the start of week 7 for 10 days, after which envelope 3 was restarted. Ingredients in envelopes provide diverse beneficial effects [24–27] (see Figure 2).

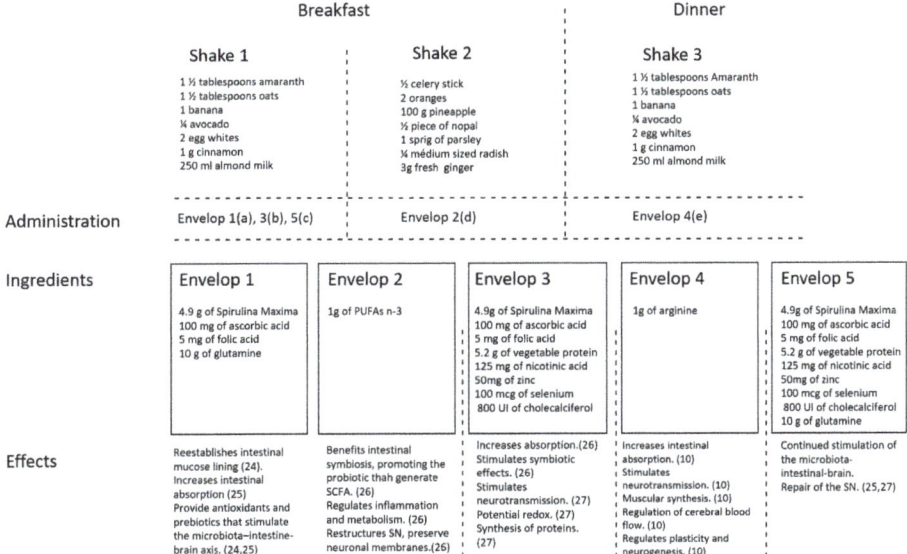

Figure 2. Schematic overview of ingredients, administration, and expected function of shakes and envelopes. (a) Administered only the first 10 days of therapy; (b) administered from day 11 until the end of week 6, after which it was suspended and substituted for envelope 5 (10 days), and then, it was retaken until the end of the intervention; (c) administered only during 10 days after the 6th week of therapy, after which envelope 3 was restarted; (d) administered throughout the intervention; (e) administered from day 8 until the end of intervention.

The total supplementation provides 287.28 kcal, 39.92 g of protein, 20 g of carbohydrates, and 4.96 g of lipids. The micronutrients that it provides are 3.81 g of fiber, 207.58 mg of sodium, 194 mg of calcium, 155 mg of phosphorus, 76 mg of magnesium, 6 mg of iron, 228.8 mg of potassium, 141.28 mg of zinc, 400 µg of selenium, 600 mg of vitamin A, 420 mg of vitamin C, 1600IU of vitamin D, 2.16 mg of vitamin E, 3.58 mg of vitamin B1, 0.76 mg of vitamin B2, 288.5 mg of vitamin B3, 8.81 mg of vitamin B5, 0.12 mg of vitamin B6, and 0.04 mg of vitamin B12.

2.5. Follow up

The participants attended the CRIT twice a week to receive physical therapy and once a week for a clinical and nutritional review. In the nutritional review every week with the parents or caregivers, it was checked that the patient had no gastrointestinal problems and that they tolerated the oral route well. Food diaries were also reviewed, and patients handed over empty supplement envelopes to verify adherence. On days the patients attended physical therapy, they were supervised to ensure that they had breakfast, a mid-morning snack, and lunch.

2.6. GMFM Assessment

The GMFM scale was performed at baseline time and weeks 7 and 13 after intervention. The evaluators and the CRIT staff were the blinded aspects of the study as they did not have access to any information about the treatment each child was receiving. The patients and their families were not blinded, so they were warned to avoid any comment on the treatment that the patient received.

This scale assesses five general parameters: 1. Lying (decubitus) and rolling over (GMFAV), 2. Sitting (GMFB), 3. Crawling and kneeling (GMFC), 4. Standing (GMFD), 5. Walking (GMFE), and one final total item (GMFF). The scoring system consists of 88 items, and each one is valued based on the following criteria: 0 = No, 1 = start, 2 = Partially Complete, 3 = Complete, NE = Not evaluated [28]. The literature has reported a high convergent validity (0.91) of the GMFCS, on GMFM [29]. Robert Palisano, the author of the scale, attended the CRIT EDO MEX to carry out training to the evaluator of this study.

2.7. Statistical Methods

In order to know the distribution of the data, the test of Shapiro–Wilk was applied. Analysis of data was performed using the Mann Whitney U test or the Kruskal Wallis followed by the Dunn posthoc test. In order to calculate the size of the effect on standing and walking evaluations, we used Rosenthal's r, an effect size test for data with non-normal distribution. This test can be used alongside Mann Whitney U-test results. The level of significance was considered as <0.05 in all cases.

2.8. Sample Size

As this investigation was an exploratory study, sample size was determined by the feasibility of recruitment. A sample of 10 children per group was established considering that the number of patients per year at CRIT—with the criteria required for the study—fluctuates between 10 and 15 patients. This sample size allows the detection of an effect size of 0.1 or larger. In order to reach the established sample, we required a three-year period.

3. Results

Fifty-three patients were interviewed. From this group, only thirty were recruited and studied from January 2015 until February 2018. The trial was stopped at this time to evaluate the preliminary results. The analysis of evaluations was made on the original assigned groups (three groups, 10 patients per group; see Figure 1). The demographic characteristics of the patients studied are summarized in Table 1.

As the adherence to the course of treatment was strictly supervised, more than 90% of patients complied with the intervention therapy. Each patient was requested to keep a food diary, which enabled us to establish their caloric intake per day. The average of kcal consumed at the start of the study in FG was 1292.5 kcal; in GC, 1495 kcal; and in IG, 1447.5 kcal. In week 13, the average kcal consumption was 1305 kcal in the FG group, 1113 kcal in CG, and 2898.8 kcal in IG.

3.1. Baseline Results

The baseline values of GMFM parameters (lying, sitting, crawling, standing, and walking) were not statistically different among the studied groups: lying (FG: 92.75 ± 3.44; CG: 93.34 ± 2.92; IG: 84.13 ± 8.87; mean ± SEM; $p = 0.950$; Kruskal Wallis followed by Dunn's posthoc test), sitting (FG: 61.34 ± 5.24; CG: 74.15 ± 5.49; IG: 75.16 ± 8.09; $p = 0.089$), crawling (FG: 49.52 ± 5.56; CG: 47.38 ± 8.90; IG: 61.86 ± 7.79; $p = 0.248$), standing (FG: 13.44 ± 3.46; CG: 15.66 ± 3.25; IG: 16.79 ± 4.58; $p = 0.666$), walking (FG: 15.49 ± 1.51; CG: 18.05 ± 1.90; IG: 20.27 ± 3.24; $p = 0.365$).

Table 1. Clinical characterization of patients with cerebral palsy (CP).

Group	Gender	Age (Years) 7.2 → 1.9	GMFD Basal Score	GMFE Basal Score
FG	F	9.6	7.7	11.4
FG	F	4.8	7.7	14.2
FG	M	5.7	7.7	18.3
FG	M	4.5	17.7	18.3
FG	M	6.8	5.1	18.3
FG	M	7.5	7.7	8.8
FG	F	5.1	27.7	25.0
FG	F	9.3	7.7	11.1
FG	M	5.5	37.7	16.7
FG	F	6.3	7.7	12.8
CG	M	9.8	23.1	16.7
CG	M	9.2	7.7	12.9
CG	F	7.3	7.7	9.2
CG	M	9.7	15.4	25.0
CG	F	7.5	38.5	29.2
CG	M	5.9	7.7	22.2
CG	M	8.1	7.7	16.7
CG	M	4.6	18.0	19.4
CG	M	12	7.7	13.9
CG	M	6.1	23.1	15.3
IG	F	7	1.0	8.3
IG	F	6.4	51.1	43.1
IG	M	11	7.7	8.3
IG	M	6.2	7.7	22.2
IG	F	6.8	7.7	18.1
IG	M	8	7.7	25.0
IG	F	5.8	18	22.2
IG	M	4.8	20.5	19.4
IG	M	7.9	25.6	25.0
IG	F	7.6	20.5	11.1

FG, follow group. CG, control group. IG, intervention group. F, female. M, male. GMFD, gross motor. Function standing. GMFE, gross motor function walking.

3.2. Lying, Sitting, and Crawling Evaluations

Throughout the follow-up, lying and sitting parameters did not show any relevant difference among the groups. In the seventh week, the groups presented very similar values. Lying: FG: 95.69 ± 4; CG: 94.89 ± 7; IG: 83.92 ± 29; mean ± SEM; $p = 0.982$; Kruskal–Wallis followed by Dunn's test. Sitting: FG: 73.83 ± 2; CG: 94.89 ± 7; IG: 83.92 ± 29; $p = 0.114$. In the 13th week, no significant difference was observed among the groups. Lying: FG: 97.63 ± 2; CG: 95.56 ± 5; IG: 89.2 ± 19; mean ± SEM; $p = 0.960$; Kruskal–Wallis followed by Dunn's test. Sitting: FG: 77.33 ± 12; CG: 83.50 ± 15; IG: 90.60 ± 16; $p = 0.082$. With respect to crawling, there was not any significant difference at the seventh week: FG: 61.30 ± 19; CG: 57.29 ± 31; IG: 76.87 ± 28; $p = 0.143$, Kruskal–Wallis followed by Dunn's test. Nevertheless, at the thirteenth week, evaluations presented a significant improvement in IG patients. Crawling: FG: 57.72 ± 17; CG: 54.38 ± 30; IG: 69.86 ± 26; $p = 0.03$, Kruskal–Wallis followed by Dunn's test.

3.3. Standing and Walking Evaluations

Figure 3 shows the comparison of the FG, CG, and IG patients in the standing parameter at 7 and 13 weeks after the intervention. A total score was considered for these evaluations. Seven weeks after intervention, IG patients presented a significant improvement in standing (26.19 ± 8.2; mean ± SD) compared with FG (10.1 ± 4.9; $p = 0.0004$, Mann Whitney U test) and CG (12.98 ± 7.2; $p = 0.003$, Mann Whitney U test) groups. In order to strengthen these results, we calculated the Rosenthal's r, a statistical assessment that evaluates the effect size (clinical efficacy of the treatment). Results showed a large size effect in the standing parameter of the IG group (r = 0.64). Thirteen weeks after intervention, the improvement continued being statistically different in IG-patients (30.90 ± 8.7) compared to FG (13.32 ± 7.4, p = 0.0002, Mann Whitney U test) and CG (17.29 ± 8.1, p = 0.003 Mann Whitney U test) groups. In this case, we also calculated Rosenthal's r and found a large effect in the IG group (r = 0.61).

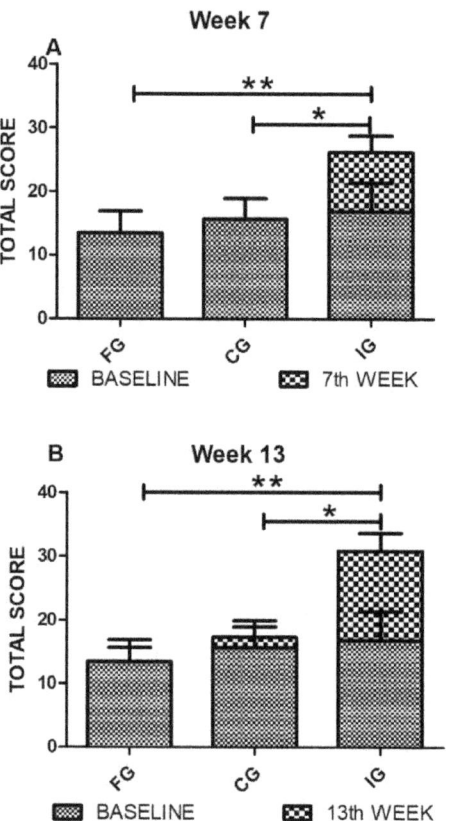

Figure 3. GMFD (standing) evaluations of FG, CG, and IG. (**A**) Standing evaluations on the seventh-week show a significant improvement of IG-patients compared to FG and CG ones. Analysis was performed by the Mann Whitney U test, * p = 0.003 ** p = 0.0004. (**B**) The standing evaluations at 13th-week show a significant improvement of the IG compared to the FG and CG groups. Analysis by the Mann Whitney U test, * p = 0.003 ** p = 0.0002. Bars represent mean ± SD of 10 patients. Baseline values are also shown.

Figure 4 shows the comparison among FG, CG, and IG patients in walking parameter at 7 and 13 weeks after the intervention. Total score was considered. Seven weeks after intervention, there was a significant difference in walking improvement in IG-patients (24.65 ± 6.1) relative to FG (18.47 ± 5.7; p = 0.01, Mann Whitney U test) and CG (19.45 ± 5.6; p = 0.03, Mann Whitney U test) ones. Rosenthal's r test showed a large effect size in the IG group (r = 0.37). After thirteen weeks, IG-patients continued presenting a significant improvement (34.68 ± 7.3) as compared to the FG (19.86 ± 6; p = 0.0003, Mann Whitney U test) and CG (22.51 ± 5.9; p = 0.001, Mann Whitney U test) patients. We also calculated Rosenthal's r for this data set. Results showed a large size effect of treatment in IG-patients on walking parameter at thirteen weeks (r = 0.67). Finally, from this group of patients (IG), five managed to walk by themselves (with no support from anyone else). No patient from the FG or CG groups achieved walking independently.

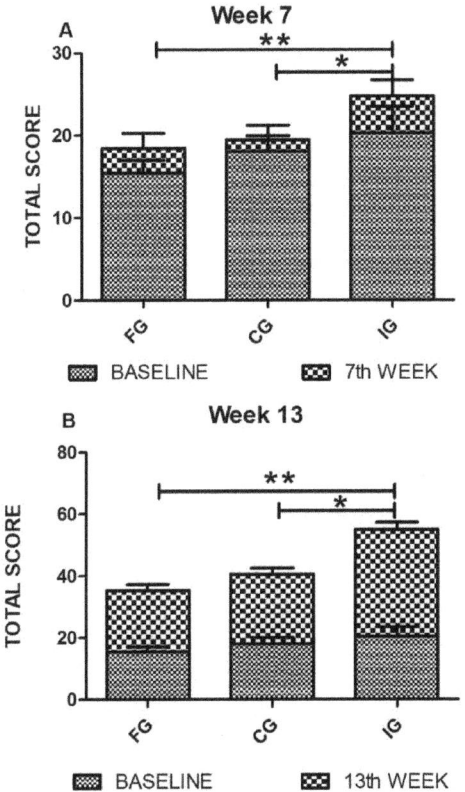

Figure 4. GMFE (walking) evaluations of FG, CG, and IG. (**A**) On the seventh week of evaluation, walking parameters showed a significant improvement in IG-patients. Analysis by the Mann Whitney U test. * $p = 0.03$ ** $p = 0.01$. (**B**) Walking evaluations on the 13th week showed a significant improvement of IG-patients compared with those of FG and CG. Analysis was performed using the Mann Whitney U test, * $p = 0.001$ ** $p = 0.0003$. Bars represent mean ± SD of 10 patients. Baseline values are also shown.

3.4. Percentage of Evolution

Figure 5 shows the comparison of the percentage of evolution in standing among the studied groups. Percentage was calculated according to the formula: final corresponding value (7 or 13 weeks)/baseline value − 1 × 100). Therefore, we are reporting the percentage of evolution after 7 or 13 weeks of intervention. IG-patients showed a significant improvement in the percentage of evolution compared to both FG and CG patients ($p = 0.025$, Kruskall Wallis followed by Dunn's posthoc test). The evolution towards the thirteenth week also revealed a significant difference in the improvement of IG-patients compared with FG and CG ones ($p = 0.03$, Kruskall Wallis followed by Dunn's posthoc test).

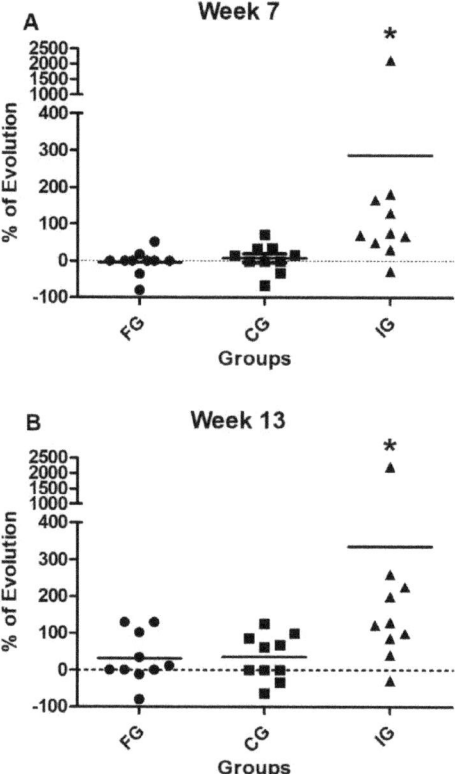

Figure 5. Percentage of evolution (GMFD, standing) of FG, CG, and IG. (**A**) The evolution from the baseline to the seventh week shows a significant improvement of standing ability in IG in comparison with the one observed in FG and CG patients. * $p = 0.025$, Kruskal Wallis test. (**B**) The evolution from the baseline towards the 13th week shows significant improvement in standing ability of IG compared to FG and CG patients. * $p = 0.03$, Kruskal Wallis test. Black line represents the mean of 10 patients.

When the walking parameter was analyzed, the evolution from the baseline to the seventh week did not present any significant advantage for any of the groups (Figure 6; $p = 0.15$, Kruskall Wallis followed by Dunn's test). Nevertheless, in the evolution observed up to the thirteenth week, IG patients presented a significant improvement, compared with FG and CG patients ($p = 0.03$, Kruskall Wallis followed by Dunn's test).

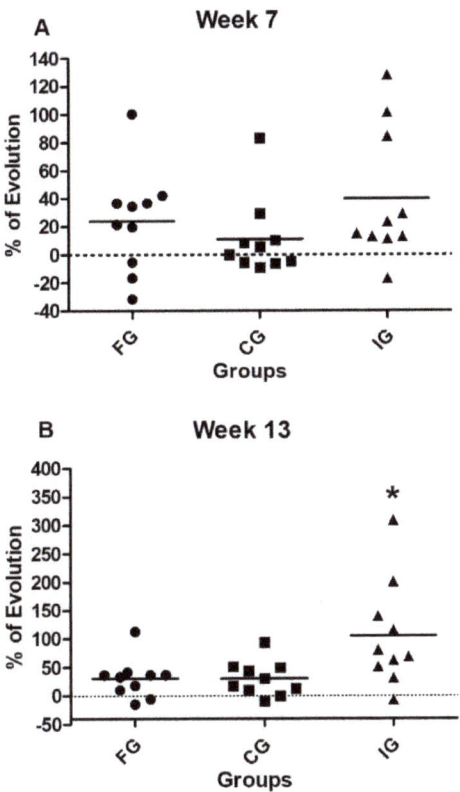

Figure 6. Percentages of evolution (GMFE, walking) of FG, CG, and IG. (**A**) The comparison of the percentages of evolution from the baseline to the seventh week does not show significant improvement in the progress of studied groups. Analysis was performed by using the Kruskal Wallis test. (**B**) The percentage of evolution from the baseline towards the 13th week shows significant improvement of the progress of IG compared to FG and CG patients., * $p = 0.029$, Kruskal Wallis test. Black line represents the mean of 10 patients.

4. Discussion

In this work, we evaluated the effect of an NSS for improving motor function in patents with CP. Our findings showed that the NSS promoted a significant improvement in standing and walking parameters of the GMFM scale. Moreover, NSS-therapy caused half of the patients studied to walk by themselves. This is a relevant finding since the improvement in motor function was, in a shorter time, above the one observed in patients with CP undergoing only conventional therapy [5]. From the initial evaluation (7 weeks after the onset of therapy), the performance of IG-patients was better than the one observed in CG and FG groups, which presented a performance that was similar to that reported in the literature [30]. The improvement of IG-treated patients was evident thirteen weeks after therapy initiation. The results observed in IG-treated patients went beyond the ones reported before using only physical therapy (2–3% of annual advance) [5]. It is of relevance to mention that even though the baseline values of IG-patients were slightly higher, the difference among the groups was not statistically significant. In order to avoid any confusion on this matter, we performed an analysis of the percentage of improvement among the different groups (this analysis included the baseline values). Therefore, we are reporting the percentage of evolution after 7 or 13 weeks of intervention. The analysis confirmed that the results were not influenced by the baseline values.

The encouraging outcome of IG-treated patients could be due to the administration of diverse nutrients and supplements that are necessary in order to compensate the metabolic, nutritional, and neurological deficiencies presented by patients with CP.

Neurological patients regularly present an increased catabolism [31]; however, in some investigations, it is reported that some patients, especially those with CP, present a lower energy requirement than healthy patients although specific nutritional information, including proteins, is not known [32]. It was observed during this investigation that the energy consumption in the baseline of all the groups was around 1300 to 1400 kcal, and the nutriments intake increased in the IG patients around 2890 kcal per day on the 13th week, being the double of kcal intake in comparison with the other groups. It is likely that after deworming, supplementing, and consuming a specific diet, they were able to increase their calorie consumption. The NSS was the only different variable among the groups. Therefore, NSS could be—at least in part—the cause of this increment. Nevertheless, other factors—non-identified at this moment—could also be participating. Further studies should be designed to corroborate these results, find other possible factors, and to establish new nutritional recommendations in CP.

The observed improvements in standing and walking can be related to a reduction in spasticity. Changes were also observed in hand movements in the majority of IG patients, which resulted in the release of the thumb and pincer grip from the "claw hand". Spasticity is related to a lesion in the Pyramidal System (PS); therefore, any improvement in these areas can be associated with a remodeling of the PS and thereby, of the CNS—in particular, in the areas of motor and premotor cortex as well as brainstem. This remodeling could be related with myelination, neurogenesis, promotion of release in neurotransmitters, or even the generation of ganglia [30]. The PS is made up of approximately one million fibers—mainly myelinated whose origins are in the primary motor and premotor cortex (80% of the fibers). Their function is to control voluntary movements, both fine and gross motor skills, in such a way that any alteration in these fibers can cause, amongst other alterations, spasticity [33].

Therefore, any therapy based on PS remodeling could be contributing to diminished spasticity and thereby, to improve fine and gross motor skills in patients with CP.

The induction or increment of plasticity phenomena, or even of regenerating neurons by providing substrates as nutrients, is extremely viable. A number of different nutrients, such as PUFAs n-3 (EPA and DHA), have been employed separately to stimulate plasticity and new neuronal cell bodies [30]. Nutrients such as zinc, ascorbic acid, spirulina, arginine, PUFAs n-3, and vitamin D have all been used in the repair of neuronal cell bodies and in neuronal regeneration [34,35]. Nevertheless, there is no scientific evidence from studies using an integrative nutritional support as a therapeutic strategy in CNS diseases. Moreover, investigations combining at least 3 or more nutrients are not available in the scientific literature.

On the other hand, it is known that the production of neurotransmitters such as serotonin and GABA can be increased using probiotics, nicotinic acid, cobalamine, pyridoxine, folates, zinc, ascorbic acid, and triptofane [36]. Regulating the production of serotonin and GABA can help to control spasticity and thus, fine and gross motor functions. The use of probiotics has become relevant in improving signaling from the intestine and favoring neurotransmission, metabolism, immunity, and inflammation through stimulating the microbiota-gut-brain axis [37].

Recently, studies on gut microbiota have become relevant in the treatment of various neurological disorders, including autism, alterations in memory, and neuronal regeneration [11]. It is also known that simultaneous supplementation of pro and prebiotics, such as inuline and other nutrients such as glutamine, induce the generation of short chain fatty acids which modulate inflammation and favor regeneration of the nervous system [38] as well as reestablishing enterocytes and muscular synthesis [39].

Finally, studies in mice showed that glutamine together with probiotics inhibit nitric oxide, reducing levels of proinflammatory factors such as TNF alfa, IL6, IL8, and reactive oxygen species

(ROS) [40]. The evidence demonstrates that combining probiotics with other nutrients to create symbiosis induces positive effects on immunity, reestablishing mucose and the nervous system.

Although the results of this investigation are encouraging, it is important to consider the constraints of the study. Perhaps the main limitation of this work is the number of evaluated patients. In the present investigation, we could not gather more than 10 individuals per group. This was mainly because the patients did not meet the inclusion criteria. The use of other therapeutic alternatives (i.e., botulinum toxin or muscle relaxants) is very common in patients with CP, and this did not allow us to include them into the study. Further research needs to be undertaken in a larger sample to support the preliminary findings of this study. Additionally, we will implement evaluations such as anthropometry, electromyography, and gait and movement analysis.

On the other hand, it is important to carry out this investigation in a research center with a controlled system, where children and their caregivers could coexist closely during the 13 weeks of the protocol. Finally, despite the convincing clinical findings, it is important to complement further research with sensitive analytical methods to evaluate neuroregeneration or neurogenesis.

Regardless of all these constraints, our findings deserve to be considered for future investigations, since they are the result of a well-controlled and designed study, which, by nature, can be replicated and carried out in other populations. Additionally, the results of this study indicate a positive relationship between NSS and gross motor skills in CP. This means that children with CP who have high-energy supplementary foods, combined with micronutrients in special doses, will further improve gross motor skills. Ati et al. [41] reported similar observations: they found a significant relationship between nutritional status and gross motor children's development. Finally, it is worth mentioning that in this investigation, nutrition was used as a stimulus to repair the nervous system—specifically, the pyramidal system. This is an innovative strategy with no previous similar studies. This exploratory investigation managed to induce better gross motor recovery in a shorter period of time as compared to conventional treatment.

Future studies should be directed to expand and confirm the results of this study.

5. Conclusions

Together, the results of this investigation provide insights into the positive effect of NSS on CP. We speculate that the observed results are mainly a consequence of a significant reduction in spasticity, which could be the result, at least in part, of a PS remodeling. In this scenario, the effect of all of the NSS components is crucial; however, we consider that the participation of PUFAs, zinc, ascorbic acid, spirulina, or arginine could be critical to repair neural function.

Author Contributions: Conceptualization, F.L.-M., M.L.-A., and A.I.; data curation, F.L.-M.; formal analysis, A.I.; funding acquisition, F.L.-M. and A.I.; investigation, F.L.-M., F.C.-S., and A.A.E.-E.; methodology, F.L.-M., D.F., and A.P.-R.; project administration, F.L.-M., X.D.L., and M.L.-E.; resources, A.I.; supervision, O.G.R.-L.; writing—review and editing, F.L.-M. and A.I. All authors have read and agreed to the published version of the manuscript.

Funding: This research was partially funded by the Centro de Investigación en Ciencias de la Salud (CICSA), FCS, Universidad Anáhuac Campus Norte, grant number 2014/03001; Valdecasas Laboratorios y Alimentos Esenciales para la Humanidad. The funders had no role in study design, data collection, and analysis, decision to publish, or preparation of the manuscript.

Acknowledgments: We would like to thank the authorities at Centro de Rehabilitación e Inclusión Infantil Teletón (CRIT) for lending us their facilities and their staff, the students who gave their time, and Keri Craig for helping to review this article.

Conflicts of Interest: The authors declare no conflict of interest. The funders had no role in the design of the study; in the collection, analyses, or interpretation of data; in the writing of the manuscript, or in the decision to publish the results.

References

1. Calzada-Vázquez-Vela, C.; Vidal-Ruiz, C.A. Parálisis cerebral infantil: Definición y clasificación a través de la historia. *Rev. Mex. Ortop. Pediátr.* **2014**, *16*, 6–10.
2. Camacho-Salas, A.; Pallás-Alonso, C.R.; de la Cruz-Bértolo, J.; Heras, R.S.D.L.; Beato, F.M. Parálisis cerebral: Concepto y registros de base poblacional. *Rev. Neurol.* **2007**, *45*, 503–508. [CrossRef] [PubMed]
3. Honeycutt, A.; Grosse, S.; Dunlap, L.; Schendel, D.E.; Chen, H.; Brann, E.; al Homsi, G. Economic costs of mental retardation, cerebral palsy, hearing loss and vision impairment—United States 2003. Centers for Disease Control and Prevention. *Morb. Mortal. Wkly. Rep.* **2004**, *53*, 57–59.
4. Rosenbaum, P.; Paneth, N.; Leviton, A.; Goldstein, M.; Bax, M.; Damiano, D.; Dan, B.; Jacobsson, B. A report: The definition and classification of cerebral palsy April 2006. *Dev. Med. Neurol. Suppl.* **2007**, *109*, 8–14.
5. Cejane-Oliveira-Martins, P.; Barbosa, M.A.; Celeno-Porto, C. Relación entre la calidad de vida de madres de niños con parálisis cerebral y la función motora de los niños, después de diez meses de rehabilitación. *Rev. Lat.-Am. Enferm.* **2010**, *18*, 149–155.
6. Krick, J.; Murphy, P.E.; Markham, J.F.; Shapiro, B.K. A proposed formula for calculating energy needs of children with cerebral palsy. *Dev. Med. Child Neurol.* **1992**, *34*, 481–487. [CrossRef]
7. Cobo, E.A.; Quino, A.C.; Díaz, D.M.; Chacón, M.J. Escala Gross Motor Function Measure. Una revisión de la literatura. *Rev. Cienc. Salud* **2014**, *2*, 11–21.
8. Herrera-Anaya, E.; Angarita-Fonseca, A.; Herrera-Galindo, V.M.; Martínez-Marín, R.D.P.; Rodríguez-Bayona, C.N. Association between gross motor function and nutritional status in children with cerebral palsy: A cross-sectional study from Colombia. *Dev. Med. Child Neurol.* **2016**, *58*, 936–941. [CrossRef]
9. Bell, K.L.; Samson-Fang, L. Nutritional management of children with cerebral palsy. *Eur. J. Clin. Nutr.* **2013**, *67*, S13–S16. [CrossRef]
10. Virarkar, M.; Alappat, L.; Bradford, P.G.; Awad, A.B. L-arginine and nitric oxide in CNS function and neurodegenerative diseases. *Crit. Rev. Food Sci. Nutr.* **2013**, *53*, 1157–1167. [CrossRef]
11. Rotstein, N.P.; Politi, L.E.; German, O.L.; Girotti, R. Protective Effect of Docosahexaenoic Acid on Oxidative Stress-Induced Apoptosis of Retina Photoreceptors. *Investig. Ophthalmol. Vis. Sci.* **2003**, *44*, 2252–2259. [CrossRef] [PubMed]
12. Pu, H.; Jiang, X.; Hu, X.; Xia, J.; Hong, D.; Zhang, W.; Gao, Y.; Chen, J.; Shi, Y. Delayed Docosahexaenoic Acid Treatment Combined with Dietary Supplementation of Omega-3 Fatty Acids Promotes Long-Term Neurovascular Restoration After Ischemic Stroke. *Transl. Stroke Res.* **2016**, *7*, 521–534. [CrossRef] [PubMed]
13. Zhang, W.; Wang, H.; Zhang, H.; Leak, R.K.; Shi, Y.; Hu, X.; Gao, Y.; Chen, J. Dietary supplementation with omega-3 polyunsaturated fatty acids robustly promotes neurovascular restorative dynamics and improves neurological functions after stroke. *Exp. Neurol.* **2003**, *272*, 170–180. [CrossRef] [PubMed]
14. Romo-Araiza, A.; Gutiérrez-Salmeán, G.; Galván, E.J.; Hernández-Frausto, M.; Herrera-López, G.; Romo-Parra, H.; García-Contreras, V.; Fernández-Presas, A.M.; Jasso-Chávez, R.; Borlongan, C.V.; et al. Probiotics and prebiotics as a therapeutic strategy to improve memory in a model of middle-aged rats. *Front. Aging Neurosci.* **2018**, *10*, 416. [CrossRef] [PubMed]
15. Zamudio-Vázquez, V.P.; Ramírez-Mayans, J.A.; Toro-Monjaraz, E.M.; Cervantes-Bustamante, R.; Zarate-Mondragon, F.; Montijo-Barrios, E.; Cadena-León, J.F.; Cázares-Méndez, J.M. Importance of gastrointestinal microbiota in children. *Acta Pediátr. México* **2017**, *38*, 49–62. [CrossRef]
16. Chen, J.; Xia, H.E.; Duan, Y.; Peng, Y.; Zhang, M. Metabolic Profile of Dyskinetic Cerebral Palsy Based on Metabonomics. *Chin. J. Rehabil. Theory Pract.* **2016**, *22*, 448–454.
17. Hillesund, E.; Skranes, J.; Trygg, K.U.; Bøhmer, T. Micronutrient status in children with cerebral palsy. *Acta Paediatr.* **2007**, *96*, 1195–1198. [CrossRef]
18. Baer, M.T.; Kozlowski, B.W.; Blyler, E.M.; Trahms, C.M.; Taylor, M.L.; Hogan, M.P. Vitamin D, calcium and bone status in children with developmental delay in relation to anti-convulsant use and ambulatory status. *Am. J. Clin. Nutr.* **1997**, *65*, 1042–1051. [CrossRef]
19. Henderson, R.; Lark, R.; Gurka, M.; Worley, G.; Fung, E.B.; Conaway, M.; Stallings, V.A.; Stevenson, R.D. Bone density and metabolism in children and adolescents with moderate to severe cerebral palsy. *Pediatrics* **2002**, *110*, 5. [CrossRef]

20. Affan, M.A.; Lee, D.W.; Al-Harbi, S.M.; Kim, H.-J.; Abdulwassi, N.I.; Heo, S.-J.; Oh, C.; Park, H.-S.; Ma, C.W.; Lee, H.-Y.; et al. Variation of Spirulina maxima biomass production in different depths of urea-used culture medium. *Braz. J. Microbiol.* **2015**, *46*, 991–1000. [CrossRef]
21. Intestinal Parasites: Control Strategies. Available online: http://www.who.int/ctd/intpara/strategies.htlm (accessed on 22 July 2020).
22. Nieuwoudt, C.H. Nutrition in neurological disability in paediatrics: Cerebral palsy. *S. Afr. J. Clin. Nutr.* **2012**, *25*, 73–76. [CrossRef]
23. World Healt Organization. mhGAP Intervention. Guide for Mental, Neurological and Substance Use Disorders in Non-Specialized Health Setting. Available online: https://www.who.int/mental_health/publications/mhGAP_intervention_guide/en/ (accessed on 12 July 2020).
24. Wang, B.; Wu, G.; Zhou, Z.; Dai, Z.; Sun, Y.; Ji, Y.; Li, W.; Wang, W.; Liu, C.; Han, F.; et al. Glutamine and intestinal barrier function. *Amino Acids* **2015**, *47*, 2143–2154. [CrossRef] [PubMed]
25. Patel, S.; Goyal, A. The current trends and future perspectives of prebiotics research: A review. *3 Biotech* **2012**, *2*, 115–125. [CrossRef]
26. Dyall, S.C. Long-chain omega-3 fatty acids and the brain: A review of the independent and shared effects of EPA, DPA and DHA. *Front. Aging Neurosci.* **2015**, *7*, 42. [CrossRef] [PubMed]
27. Siegel, G.J.; Agranoff, B.W.; Albers, R.W.; Fisher, S.K.; Uhler, M.D. *Basic Neurochemistry: Molecular, Cellular and Medical Aspects*, 6th ed.; Lippincott-Raven: Philadelphia, PA, USA, 1999.
28. Wood, E.; Rosenbaun, P. The Gross Motor Function Classification System for cerebral palsy. *Dev. Med. Child Neurol.* **2000**, *42*, 292–296. [CrossRef]
29. Bodkin, A.W.; Robinson, C.; Perales, F.P. Reliability and Validity of the Gross Motor Function Classification System for Cerebral Palsy. *Pediatr. Phys. Ther.* **2003**, *15*, 247–252. [CrossRef]
30. Ohata, K.; Tsuboyama, T.; Haruta, T.; Ichihashi, N.; Kato, T.; Nakamura, T. Relation between muscle thickness, spasticity, and activity limitations in children and adolescents with cerebral palsy. *Dev. Med. Child Neurol.* **2008**, *50*, 152–156. [CrossRef]
31. Hogan, S.E. Energy requirements of children with cerebral palsy. *Can. J. Diet. Pract. Res.* **2004**, *65*, 124–130. [CrossRef]
32. García-Contreras, A.A.; Vásquez-Garibay, E.M.; Romero-Velarde, E.; Ibarra-Gutiérrez, A.I.; Troyo-Sanromán, R. Energy expenditure in children with cerebral palsy and moderate/severe malnutrition during nutritional recovery. *Nutr. Hosp* **2015**, *31*, 2062–2069.
33. Salazar, Z.A. Neurogénesis y actividad física. *Rev. Neurol. Neurocir. Psiquiatr.* **2004**, *37*, 167–170.
34. Le Roy, C.; Rebollo, M.J.; Moraga, M.F.; Sm, X.D. Castillo-Durán, C.Nutrición del niño con enfermedades neurológicas prevalentes. *Rev. Chil. Pediatr.* **2010**, *81*, 110–113.
35. Planas, M. Metabolic-nutritional aspects in neurological diseases. *Nutr. Hosp.* **2014**, *29*, 3–12.
36. Ehninger, D.; Kempermann, G. Neurogenesis in the adult hippocampus. *Cell Tissue Res.* **2008**, *331*, 243–250. [CrossRef]
37. Fernández, R.M.; Rodríguez, L.I.; López-Ibor, A.M. Suplementos nutricionales en el trastorno de ansiedad. *Actas Esp. Psiquiatr.* **2017**, *45*, 1–7.
38. Mangiola, F.; Ianiro, G.; Franceschi, F.; Fagiuoli, S.; Gasbarrini, G.; Gasbarrini, A. Gut microbiota in autism and mood disorders. *World J. Gastroenterol.* **2016**, *22*, 361–368. [CrossRef] [PubMed]
39. Alkasir, R.; Li, J.; Li, X.; Jin, M.; Zhu, B. Human gut microbiota: The links with dementia development. *Protein Cell* **2016**, *8*, 90–102. [CrossRef] [PubMed]
40. Borre, Y.E.; O'Keeffe, G.W.; Clarke, G.; Stanton, C.; Dinan, T.G.; Cryan, J.F. Microbiota and neurodevelopmental windows: Implications for brain disorders. *Trends Mol. Med.* **2014**, *20*, 509–518. [CrossRef] [PubMed]
41. Ati, C.A.; Alfiyanti, D.; Solekhan, A. Hubungan Antara Status Gizi Dengan Perkembangan Motorik Kasar Anak Balita Di RSUD Tugurejo Semarang Tahun. *J. Ilmu Keperawatan Dan Kebidanan* **2013**, *33*, 1–8.

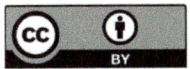

© 2020 by the authors. Licensee MDPI, Basel, Switzerland. This article is an open access article distributed under the terms and conditions of the Creative Commons Attribution (CC BY) license (http://creativecommons.org/licenses/by/4.0/).

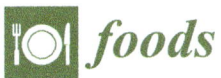

Article

The Effect of L-Theanine Incorporated in a Functional Food Product (Mango Sorbet) on Physiological Responses in Healthy Males: A Pilot Randomised Controlled Trial

Jackson Williams [1], Andrew J. McKune [1,2,3], Ekavi N. Georgousopoulou [4,5,6], Jane Kellett [1], Nathan M. D'Cunha [1], Domenico Sergi [7], Duane Mellor [8] and Nenad Naumovski [1,*]

1. Faculty of Health, University of Canberra, Canberra, ACT 2601, Australia; jackson.williams@canberra.edu.au (J.W.); andrew.mckune@canberra.edu.au (A.J.M.); jane.kellett@canberra.edu.au (J.K.); nathan.dcunha@canberra.edu.au (N.M.D)
2. Discipline of Biokinetics, Exercise and Leisure Sciences, School of Health Sciences, University of KwaZulu-Natal, Durban, KwaZulu-Natal 4000, South Africa
3. Research Institute of Sport and Exercise, University of Canberra, Canberra, ACT 2605, Australia
4. Centre for Health and Medical Research, ACT Health Directorate, Canberra, ACT 2601, Australia; ekavigeorgousopoulou@gmail.com
5. Medical School, Australian National University, Canberra, ACT 2601, Australia
6. School of Medicine, University of Notre Dame Australia, Sydney, NSW 2000, Australia
7. Nutrition & Health Substantiation Group, Nutrition and Health Program, Health and Biosecurity, Commonwealth Scientific and Industrial Research Organisation (CSIRO), Adelaide, SA 5000, Australia; Domenico.Sergi@csiro.au
8. Aston Medical School, Aston University, Birmingham B47ET, UK; d.mellor@aston.ac.uk
* Correspondence: nenad.naumovski@canberra.edu.au

Received: 27 February 2020; Accepted: 18 March 2020; Published: 23 March 2020

Abstract: Consumption of L-Theanine (L-THE) has been associated with a sensation of relaxation, as well as a reduction of stress. However, these physiological responses have yet to be elucidated in humans where L-THE is compared alongside food or as a functional ingredient within the food matrix. The aim of this study was to determine the physiological responses of a single intake of a potential functional food product (mango sorbet) containing L-THE (ms-L-THE; 200 mgw/w) in comparison to a flavour and colour-matched placebo (ms). Eighteen healthy male participants were recruited in this randomised, double-blind, placebo-controlled trial. The participants were required to consume ms-L-THE or placebo and their blood pressure (BP) (systolic and diastolic), heart rate (HR), and heart rate variability (HRV) were monitored continuously over 90 minutes. Eleven males (age 27.7 ± 10.8 years) completed the study. Changes in area under the curve for systolic and diastolic blood pressure and HRV over the 90 minute observation period indicated no differences between the three conditions (all $p > 0.05$) or within individual groups (all $p > 0.05$). The values for heart rate were also not different in the placebo group ($p = 0.996$) and treatment group ($p = 0.066$), while there was a difference seen at the baseline ($p = 0.003$). Based on the findings of this study, L-THE incorporated in a food matrix (mango sorbet) demonstrated no reduction in BP or HR and showed no significant parasympathetic interaction as determined by HRV high-frequency band and low-frequency/high-frequency ratio. Further studies should be focussed towards the comparison of pure L-THE and incorporation within the food matrix to warrant recommendations of L-THE alongside food consumption.

Keywords: L-Theanine; amino acid; green tea; bioactive; functional food; blood pressure; heart rate variability; cardiometabolic effect

1. Introduction

Stress is a dynamic condition that acts as a stimulus, affecting arousal factors of individuals in response to challenges and aversive situations. The consequences of stress are strongly influenced by how an individual perceives and appraises the situation in addition to the intensity of the event that triggers the stress response [1–3]. Traditionally, consumption of tea is associated with relaxation [3], beneficial health outcomes [4], and an increase in longevity, which is proposed to be due to a number of different bioactive constituents [5,6]. Prior to its consumption, tea leaves undergo processing and based on the type of processing, predominantly leads to seven different types of tea; 'green' (unfermented), 'yellow', 'white', 'oolong' (partially fermented), 'black' (completely fermented), 'aged pu-erh' (drastically fermented and aged), and 'ripened pu-erh' tea [7]. The type of processing also affects the formation of different compounds, including but not limited to the composition and degradation of the molecules found in green tea. In green tea, the steaming (or heating) process inactivates the enzyme polyphenol oxidase, which prevents the further fermentation of tea leaves, consequently producing a stable and dry product. During this process, oxidative polymerisation of monomeric flavan-3-ols is inhibited (unlike in the black and other teas), and green tea typically contains higher levels of these flavan-3-ols. Therefore, it can be anticipated that different processing techniques will also influence the levels of other molecules and putative bioactives, such as amino acids.

Derived from the leaves of the *Camellia sinensis* species, green tea is consumed due to its favourable taste and also for its reported therapeutic properties such as cardiovascular benefits, increased relaxation effects and strong, anti-inflammatory [8] and antioxidant effects [6,7,9]. These effects are linked to its many bioactive constituents, including polyphenols [10], particularly catechins [11], and γ-glutamylethylamide, commonly referred to as L-Theanine (L-THE), which is the most abundant and unique non-proteinogenic amino acid in green tea.

The consumption of L-THE is associated with a sensation of relaxation, and is proposed to elicit acute stress-reducing effects [3] as well as providing the characteristic *'umami'* flavour [6]. In addition, the consumption of L-THE is associated with antihypertensive [12,13], anti-inflammatory properties [8] as well as improvements in cognitive functioning in healthy adults [14] and when consumed in combination with caffeine [10]. Studies report stress lowering effects, expressed physiologically in the form of reductions in heart rate (HR), observed post-completion of a stress-inducing mental arithmetic task after the consumption of L-THE (200 mg) in its relatively pure form [15]. Furthermore, reductions in salivary cortisol post L-THE consumption indicate the putative involvement of L-THE in hypothalamic-pituitary-adrenal (HPA) axis responses have also been reported [15,16].

The autonomic nervous system (ANS), consisting of the sympathetic nervous system (SNS) and parasympathetic nervous systems (PNS) [17,18], are of central importance to the homeostatic stress response. Blood pressure is a physiological biomarker that is highly dependant on catecholaminergic neurons [19]. The HR is also considered to be a vital indicator of the stress response, however, the changes in interval between the highest points (R-R interval) of the heartbeat observed on the electrocardiogram (usually referred to as QRS complex), known as heart rate variability (HRV), is becoming a reliable marker for the responses caused by internal and external stressors. Changes in HRV, representing ANS cardiac regulation, can be directly (*via* ANS innervation of the myocardium) or humorally (catecholamines related hormones) mediated [20]. The high frequency (HF) component of HRV ranges from 0.15-0.4 Hz, and is based on respiratory sinus arrhythmia and mediated predominantly by PNS activity, whereas low frequency (LF) ranges between 0.04-0.15 Hz, is mediated by both PNS and SNS [21]. Furthermore, the state of being stressed affects HRV domains such as HF, LF and LF/HF ratios, which are used to understand the activity of the PNS and further as an index of autonomic balance [22].

It is proposed that the 'healthier' the ANS, the better an individual will be able to exhibit high allostatic resilience [23]. As such, HRV changes are reported to be a potential marker of the relationship between food consumption and disease [24]. These findings were further supported in studies where certain components of dietary intake are associated with higher HRV, for instance the Mediterranean diet, which consists highly of fish and omega-3 fatty acid consumption, fresh produce, [25] as well as healthy weight maintenance [26] all contribute to the potential increase in HRV. On the other hand, reduced HRV is associated with an increased risk for a range of diseases including but not limited to cardiovascular disease [27] and diabetes [28]. This contributes to the possibility that HRV markers provide a fast and convenient way to measure the potential benefits of health status in response to various dietary interventions.

Regardless of the method of delivery of this non-proteinogenic amino acid, L-THE needs to be easily accessible and bioavailable in concentrations sufficient to produce the desired physiological effects. Human studies in which consumption of pure L-THE was provided in capsule form, indicate the most physiologically relevant doses of L-THE range from 0.05–0.4 g, equivalent to a consumption of 2–15 cups of green tea [6,29,30]. One method to deliver these dosages of L-THE is via the integration of pure L-THE in the food matrix as a potential functional food product. Based on the findings of our previous review [6], we propose that incorporating 200 mg of L-THE in a functional food product will provide a convenient and palatable delivery method of a physiologically relevant dose of L-THE. Therefore, the aim of this study was to determine the physiological responses HR, HRV, and blood pressure (BP) in healthy males following the one-off acute ingestion of a potential functional food product (mango sorbet) containing 200 mg of pure L-THE.

2. Methods and Materials

2.1. Participants

Participants were informed about the study protocols, provided written consent, and then screened to determine eligibility for participation. Following previously conducted research using similar design and products [11], inclusion criteria included healthy male participants aged 18–65 years old. Participants were excluded from participating if they consume: any functional foods including stanol or sterol ester-containing margarines; weight loss supplements, or commercial dietary products associated with weight loss; currently had or have had any known active pulmonary, hematologic, hepatic, gastrointestinal, renal, premalignant, malignant illnesses; have diabetes (type 1 and type 2); or any thyroid dysfunction.

2.2. Procedure

A randomised, double-blind, placebo-controlled, crossover design was used to determine the acute physiological HR, HRV, and BP effects after consumption of mango sorbet containing L-THE (200 mg). This study was approved by the Human Research Ethics Committee of the University of Canberra (HREC-193-2018) and written informed consent was obtained from all participants.

Participants were required to attend four clinic visits (Figure 1), initial screening (clinic 1), a baseline measurements clinic (clinic 2) to familiarise participants, and two blinded food consumption clinics (clinics 3 and 4). In the last two clinics, participants consumed the 100 g of the food products mango sorbet, one a placebo without active ingredient (ms) or the treatment mango sorbet containing 200 mg of L-THE (ms-L-THE). The findings from animal studies suggested that L-THE brain levels are increased 30–60 minutes post-consumption. Thus, assessment of the physiological parameters mentioned below occurred immediately post L-THE food product consumption to capture the period and curve at which L-THE exerts its effects.

Allocated randomised treatment sequences were achieved using 4 blocks of random sequencing numbers per intervention (randomizer.org) to ensure the ms and ms-L-THE sorbets administrations were balanced between the participants. The sequence code was placed in a sealed envelope and revealed only at the end of the trial once all participants finalised all of their visits. A 48 h washout period was used between clinics 3 and 4 ensuring the adequate time for the L-THE clearance from the body [29]. Prior to attending clinics 2, 3, and 4, participants were required to fast overnight (at least 8

h) except for water consumption. Participants were also asked to refrain from alcohol for 24 h, and caffeine 12 h prior the commencement of the clinic.

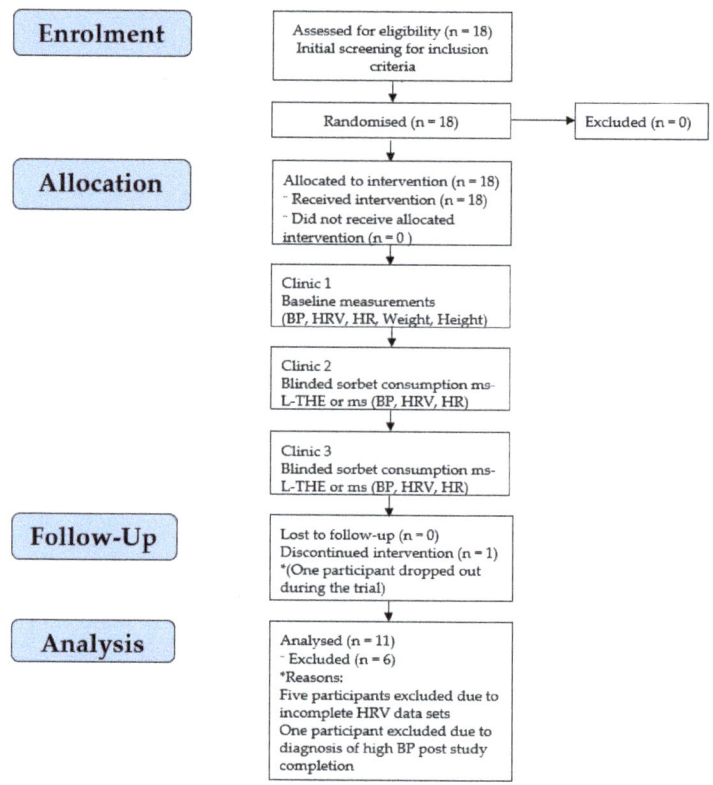

Figure 1. Consort flowchart of clinics attended in the study for the 11 included participants.

2.3. Materials and Reagents

The mango sorbet used in this study was developed based on the modified formulation described elsewhere [11]. Common mangos (Mango pieces, Coles Pty Ltd, Peru/Mexico), caster sugar (CSR, Yarraville, VIC, Australia), were purchased from local commercial suppliers. The L-THE (Suntheanine™, Taiyo Kagaku Co., Ltd, Yokkaichi Japan) was purchased from Ingredient Resources Australia and New Zealand Pty/Ltd (Sydney, NSW, Australia) and was the functional additive (200 mg/100 g w/w) to the active product. The whey protein concentrate (WPC) was purchased from Professional Whey Pty/Ltd (Erina, NSW, Australia) and added to provide structural stability and rigidity to the food product. The sorbet was selected as the food matrix of choice for this study due to the preference for storage stability of L-THE such as low temperature (less than 4 °C) and stability in an acidic environment (pH range 5–6) [31]. The dosage of L-THE (200 mg) was selected based on the findings of previous studies [29]. The nutritional composition of the ms-L-THE (Table 1), including the macro- and micronutrient data were analysed using the Australian Food Composition Database integrated into the FoodWorks Professional Software (v9, Xyris Software, Brisbane, QLD, Australia).

Table 1. Nutrient profile of the mango sorbet with L-Theanine per single serve (100 g).

Average Quantity	Per Serve (100 g)
Energy (kJ)	587
Protein (g)	8.33
Total fat (g)	<1
SATURATED (g)	<1
Carbohydrate (g)	28.07
SUGARS (g)	26.1
Fibre (g)	1.2
Sodium (mg)	15.55
L-Theanine (mg)	200

The total nutrient profile for the mango sorbet containing the active ingredient L-Theanine (L-THE) expressed as a per 100 g serve. note the mango sorbet (ms) did not contain 200 mg of L-THE.

2.4. Outcomes

2.4.1. Blood Pressure

Participants' blood pressure was determined following the guidelines for the 2nd Australian National Blood Pressure study [32]. Blood pressure was determined using the finger cuff (non-invasive BP nano, AD Instruments, Dunedin, New Zealand), using two inter-inflation cuffs that were placed on the participants in a sedentary position. Continuous readings for systolic, diastolic blood pressure were recorded, as well as inter-beat interval, HR, and mean arterial pressure over 90 minutes. The data were smoothed based on the AD instruments smoothing algorithm to remove outlying data points due to finger movement and further segmented into 18 distinct values from each 5 min interval [11].

2.4.2. Heart Rate Variability

Each participant was provided with a fitness-tracking device heart rate belt (Suunto® T6, Vantaa, Finland) that measures HR and R-R intervals of continuous electrocardiogram QRS heartbeat complexes. Participants were instructed how to use the device, ensuring the belt was placed below the chest muscles across the sternum after water was applied to the undersurface of the belt to ensure conduction [33]. Participants were required to be in a sedentary position for 10 min to establish resting measurements. During each clinic, participants were required to wear the heart rate belt in a sedentary position for the entirety of the clinic. Recordings for all clinics began after 10 minutes of participants being in a sedentary position. However, during consumption clinics, recordings began after complete consumption of each respective sorbet.

2.5. Statistical Analysis

All data obtained were analysed as a 5 min average up to 90 min. The obtained R-R interval data were downloaded from the HR monitors via the Suunto T6 Team Management Software (v2.1, Vantaa, Finland) and exported as a text file for time domain and spectral HRV analysis using the Kubios HRV Standard 3.0.2 diagnostic device software (Kuopio, Finland). All R-R interval artefacts were manually corrected using the methodology described by Sookan and McKune (2012). Using total area under the curve (AUC), the non-parametric independent samples Kruskal–Wallis ANOVA was the primary model for analysis for time effects for between-group time relationships the entire 0–90 min block, and further analysed between each 5 min period up to 90 min also using Kruskal–Wallis analysis. Both are presented as medians, 25th and 75th quartiles with Chi-square and p-value. For related samples, Friedman's two-way ANOVA by ranks was applied to test same group relationships for the entirety of 90 min, presented as Chi-square and p-value. The HF HRV values were log-transformed prior to analysis. Level of significance was set at $\alpha = 0.05$. Data were analysed using the SPSS v25 (Armonk, IBM Corp, New York, USA).

3. Results

Initially, eighteen healthy male adults were recruited with 17 completing all four study visits. Following the completion of the study, data were analysed from 11 participants (age 27.7 ± 10.8 years, weight 90.6 ± 16.8 kg) due to the following; one participant voluntarily discontinued the trial due to lost contact; data of five participants were excluded due to insufficient data points collected due to equipment malfunction, whilst one participant was excluded post-study due to a clinical diagnosis of high blood pressure. All descriptive statistics for systolic and diastolic BP, heart rate, HF HRV including 1st and 3rd quartiles, median, total AUC values described in Table 2.

Table 2. The frequencies and Area Under the Curve (AUC) of the visits for baseline, ms-L-THE, and ms sorbets consumption.

Parameters	Baseline Median (1st, 3rd Quartile) Total AUC (/90 min)	ms-L-THE Median (1st, 3rd Quartile) Total AUC (/90 min)	ms Median (1st, 3rd Quartile) Total AUC (/90 min)	p-Values Kruskal–Wallis All Visits	p-Values Friedman Baseline	p-Values Friedman ms-L-THE	p-Values Friedman ms
Systolic BP (mmHg) Total AUC (mmHg/90min)	137 (123, 151) 26776	133 (123, 143) 26160	137 (123, 148) 27043	0.839	0.147	0.853	0.990
Diastolic BP (mmHg) Total AUC (mmHg/90min)	72 (601, 88) 14717	72 (66,80) 14339	73 (62, 82) 14693	0.922	0.515	0.120	0.491
Systolic/Diastolic Total AUC (ratio/90min)	32.9 (29.4, 34.95) 33.5	31.8 (31.5, 35.7) 33.2	34.4 (30.1, 36.9) 36.0	0.970	0.761	0.003 *	0.003 *
Heart Rate (bpm) Total AUC (bpm/90min)	74 (66, 77) 14408	73, (68, 77) 14413	73 (67, 77) 14332	0.996	0.003 *	0.066	0.060
HF (Ln) HRV (Hz) Total AUC (Hz/90min)	6.22 (5.20, 6.95) 139094	6.07 (5.27, 7.16) 153344	6.38 (5.24, 7.22) 146457	0.974	0.064	0.534	0.971
LF/HF Total AUC (ratio/90min)	2.96 (2.21, 7.87) 1025	2.55 (2.06, 6.98) 905	2.60 (1.77, 5.94) 1054	0.704	0.458	0.082	0.330

The non-parametric frequencies median, 1st and 3rd quartiles and total AUC (expressed as a sum of values from the 0–90 minute period) values for systolic and diastolic BP, systolic/diastolic BP, HR, high-frequency HRV, and LF/HF HRV ratio for the 11 included participants. * Indicates significant $p < 0.05$.

3.1. Systolic and Diastolic Blood Pressure

For systolic BP, between-group analysis for AUC did not demonstrate any significant effects for the entire 90 minute period (Figure 2A) (median; 1323 mmHg, 25th; 1157 mmHg, 75th; 1462 mmHg, $p = 0.839$). Further analysis of the individual 18 × 5 minute time points showed no significant differences between the three clinic visits ($p > 0.05$). The within-group analysis provided all non-significant results respectively for the entirety of the 90 minute groups (all $p > 0.05$).

For diastolic BP, between-group AUC analysis showed no significant differences during the entirety of the 90 minutes (Figure 2B) amongst either of the conditions (median; 1323 mmHg, 25th; 1157 mmHg, 75th; 1462 mmHg, $p = 0.922$). Similarly, between-group analysis of the individual 18 × 5 minute time points also showed no significant differences between each of the three clinic visits (all $p > 0.05$). Same group analysis test indicated no significant differences within each of the conditions (all $p > 0.05$).

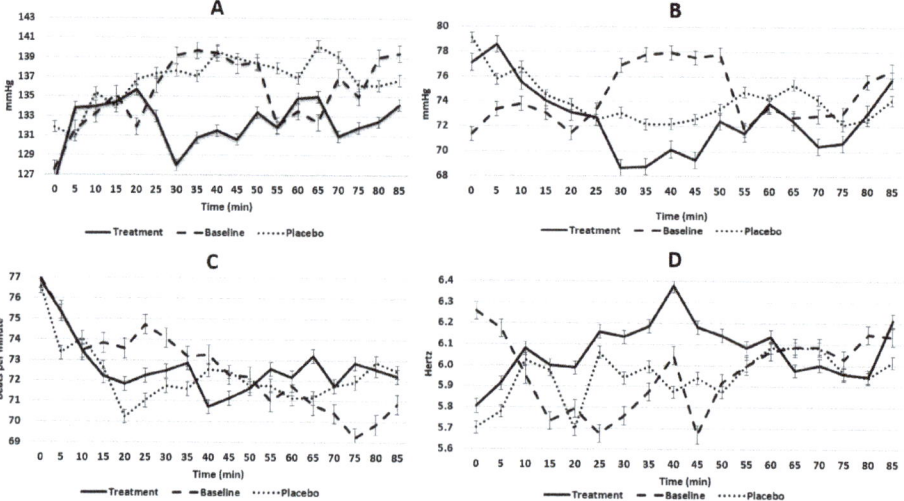

Figure 2. The changes in physiological parameters: systolic blood pressure (**A**); diastolic blood pressure (**B**), heart rate (**C**) and log of high-frequency heart rate variability (**D**) over the 90 minute period for the 11 included particpants.

3.2. Systolic/Diastolic Ratio

The ratio of systolic/diastolic AUC analysis showed no significant differences during the entirety of 90 min between either of the conditions (median; 32.3, 25th; 31.1, 75th; 35.7, $p = 0.970$). Further, analysis of the individual 18 × 5 min time points showed no significant differences between each of the three conditions (all $p > 0.05$). Same condition analysis showed no significant differences within the baseline group ($p = 0.761$), whereas significant differences were observed in the ms-L-THE group ($p = 0.003$) and the ms group ($p = 0.003$).

3.3. Heart Rate

Between-group AUC analysis showed no significant differences during the entire 90 minutes between either of the conditions (median; 1325, 25th; 1222, 75th; 1385, $p = 0.996$). Further analysis of the individual 18 × 5 min time points also showed no significant differences between each of the three conditions (all $p > 0.05$), whereas within-group analysis showed significant differences within the baseline group ($p = 0.003$) as well as within the ms-L-THE group ($p = 0.066$) (Figure 2C). No significant differences were observed in the ms group ($p = 0.060$).

3.4. Sympathetic Activity

3.4.1. High-frequency HRV

AUC HF analysis showed no significant time effects between groups (median; 97.3, 25th; 6.59, 75th; 120, $p = 0.974$). Analysis of the individual 18 × 5 min time points also showed no significant differences between each of the three conditions (all $p > 0.05$). Intergroup analysis showed no significant differences within each of the group conditions (all $p > 0.05$) (Figure 2D).

3.4.2. LF/HF Ratio

LF/HF measurements using for AUC analysis during the 90 minute period showed no significant time effects between groups (median; 50.9, 25th; 35.3, 75th; 16.3, $p = 0.704$). Analysis of the individual 18 × 5 min time points between groups showed no significant differences between each of the three conditions (all $p > 0.05$). Analysis of same group comparisons showed no significant differences within each of the group conditions (all $p > 0.05$).

4. Discussion

The current study implemented a randomised double-blind, placebo-controlled cross over design to investigate the effects of L-THE incorporated into a whey protein-based mango sorbet as a potential functional food product. To our knowledge, this study is the first to examine the effect of a functional food product containing L-THE to determine its physiological effectiveness using a continuous set of BP and HRV measurements.

The observed results for the ms-L-THE did not produce any significant physiological changes for the parameters of systolic and diastolic BP across the entire 90 minute testing period in comparison to the ms or baseline measurements. Similar to other studies where external factors such as stress or caffeine are used to raise BP, our intervention was designed to cause fluctuations in BP, HR, and HRV due to the carbohydrate response attributed to sorbet consumption [34]. Despite showing initial significant interactions, the systolic/diastolic ratio was a good indicator of the BP effect of both sorbets for within-subject effects. This indicated that consumption of both ms and ms-L-THE caused a postprandial response, in turn, causing the systolic/diastolic to show significant differences as supported by our analysis. Pharmacokinetic clinical data [35] that involved the ingestion of pure L-THE (25–200 mg) suggest peaks in physiological and blood plasma effects occur between 32 and 50 min post oral ingestion (in a fasted state) [29]. Although a similar trend is observed in our current study in terms of a time effect relationship for systolic BP reduction (Figure 2), our study design did not demonstrate any statistically significant physiological effects in comparison to the reported pharmokinetic trends that L-THE exhibits.

Further, as blood plasma concentrations were not studied in our trial, we can only speculate that the observed physiological trends in the current study are in line with the mentioned pharmacokinetic studies [29,35]. The same 200 mg L-THE dosage is clinically reported to acutely attenuate BP (the rise seen in high-stress-response adults), as well as reducing anxiety after stress loading tasks [13]. Additionally, the findings of a relatively recent study have indicated that consumption of L-THE (200 mg) has potential to promote mental health by providing better quality sleep and improvement in cognitive functioning by improving verbal fluency and executive functioning scores [14]. Similarly, a study measuring BP [36] at time points of 20 and 70 min respectively post 97 mg L-THE and 40 mg caffeine intake, highlighted the attenuative effects L-THE has on caffeine. However, this study was limited by reference of only two-time points [36]. Considering previously reported evidence regarding L-THE concentration in the blood post-consumption, it is demonstrated that L-THE potentially antagonises the BP effect of caffeine on participants, without affecting the alertness or mood aspects as well as slowing overall reaction time [37]. In the same study, the authors did not state whether a fasted state was implemented, whilst in comparison, the present study did not implement a cognitive task to raise BP and may in future benefit from an external stimulus to observe the BP effects of L-THE within the food matrix [37].

The initial results suggested that HR was significantly affected using within-subject contrasts however, further analysis revealed no significant interactions. It can be proposed that consumption of both the mango sorbet interventions stabilised HR in contrast to the significant results observed solely in the baseline clinic, however further testing by comparing L-THE in its pure form against L-THE within the food matrix must be conducted to confirm this. As such, these results fall in line with the study by Dodd et al. [10], who also reported no significant differences in HR when pure L-THE was consumed via capsule intake (50 mg); however, this may have occurred due to the low dose provided to participants. In comparison, our results were not on par with those reported by Kimura et al. [15], where consumption of 200 mg L-THE dissolved in water actively resulted in the reduction of HR in response to an acute mental arithmetic stressor task. In the design of our current study, we did not implement a mental stressor task to alter HR, and in future, may benefit from adding a mentally stressing intervention such as arithmetic task. Based on this, it is safe to say that our study is the first to identify that L-THE does not have any effect on HR when consumed within a functional food product and in the absence of environmental stressors; however, from the literature, 200 mg of pure L-THE may acutely lower HR in response to stressful situations which is thought to reflect attenuation of sympathetic nervous activation [15]. Our results do not indicate a potential for L-THE to buffer HRV physiological markers for both HF and LF/HF ratio in the periods of post-consumption. Nonetheless, the presents study suggests that L-THE did reduce the variance of HF outcomes; however, this was not shown to be statistically significant.

In humans, understanding of the physiological responses attributed to L-THE intake where pure L-THE is consumed alongside everyday foods or integrated as part of a food matrix has only been partially investigated to date. Currently, only two known studies aimed at investigating the effect of L-THE consumption embedded within food have been reported [38,39]. The first investigated a nutrient-based drink containing 200 mg of L-THE as well as alpha glycerylphosphorylcholine (α GPC; 25 mg), phosphatidylserine (1 mg), and micronised chamomile (10 mg), however, no BP or HR data was recorded and this particular study reported a decrease in salivary cortisol that supports the potential anti-stress effects of L-THE [39]. The latter study [39] displayed sympathomimetic inhibitory responses post-consumption of 128 mg L-THE within a cacao (60% w/w) chocolate that resulted in a decrease in BP associated with the L-THE condition. It has been previously suggested by Kakuda et al. [40] that the L-THE mechanism of action relies on the reduction of glutamate release from pre-synapse to the synaptic cleft by acting as an inhibitor of glutamine re-uptake. Additionally, glutamine was also associated with the replenishment of the neurotransmitter pool. This, in turn, inhibits extracellular glutamine uptake by neurons, and its conversion to glutamate via glutaminase enzyme [41]. The recent review by Yoneda et al [42] proposes a possible novel in vitro neurogenic role of L-THE for brain wellness via increase in neurogenesis. Interestingly, the findings of an animal trial using a stress-sensitive strain of mice (senescence-accelerated mice prone 10) that were exposed to stress, had decreased brain volume. However, the same strain of mice that ingested L-THE (6 mg/kg), under the same experimental conditions had a suppression in brain atrophy [43]. Although this is reported to occur based on common neuroprotective outcomes related to stress [42,43], this mechanism of action and the outcomes specific to glutamate biomarkers assessed in the Kakuda et al. [44] study were not assessed in the present study. As there were no statistically significant interactions between the baseline, ms, and ms-L-THE variables, one of the potential mechanisms that may have affected the outcomes was that the L-THE may have bound to the food matrix of the ingredients used in the sorbet (WPC, sucrose, or the mango pulp). Whilst our previous findings indicate that high-performance liquid chromatography (HPLC) analysis of the L-THE extraction from mango pulp yielded a 98% extraction (unpublished data); thus, a potential rational for the integration with mangoes, the potential for L-THE binding to the WPC or sucrose cannot be overlooked. Despite this, it is equally important to acknowledge that HPLC analysis of L-THE is unlikely to reflect the biological outcomes of L-THE in the gastrointestinal tract. Furthermore, it is difficult to determine all known bioactive constituents are present in the mango pulp as well as the WPC and sucrose, which all may affect the kinetical aspects of L-THE including but not limited to: absorption, distribution, elimination, and biotransformation. It is essential to acknowledge the unaccounted bioactive ingredients found within the mango sorbet may have lessened the effects of L-THE, however, to our knowledge, no literature suggest L-THE interacts with WPC or sucrose. Therefore, a similar study design that investigates the effects of L-THE as a mono supplement against other food matrixes is required to determine the physiological outcomes, as well as implementing techniques to monitor L-THE in the circulation as a point of reference for its bioavailability. Based on previous literature, we propose that from the results of this study, L-THE in its pure encapsulated form appears to serve as a medium for consumption to produce its known effects rather than when combined within the food matrix of mango sorbet.

Limitations and Future Directions

The lack of significant interactions observed in this study can potentially be attributed to a sample size that was reflective of the nature of this study being a pilot trial. Furthermore, due to the exclusion of data (participant exclusion), future studies should account for including a higher number of participants as well as participants with pre existing health conditions such as anxiety and high blood pressure. Furthermore, it is equally important to compare the differences between L-THE in its relatively pure form against L-THE as an integrated component of the food matrix. Although the population was male-only, we can only assume that the results are reflective of the current population included.

Further, L-THE consumed orally as a component of mango sorbet (200 mg) is a lower dose compared to the pharmacodynamic rat studies by Yokogoshi et al. [45] as well as Yokogoshi and Kobayashi [46], which were both similar in design (1500 mg/day and 2000 mg/kg of L-THE administered intraperitoneally). In future studies, administering a standardised dose adjusted for the kilograms of body weight (kg/bw) is one potential way to maximise the effects of L-THE and determine the 'ideal' and personalised dosage for healthy humans as well as potentially increasing the bioavailability of L-THE in the body. However, it is equally important to acknowledge that further research must be conducted where L-THE as a component of a functional food product is compared alongside L-THE in its pure encapsulated form to warrant any clinically relevant claims.

5. Conclusions

Our results suggest that consumption of L-THE within the functional food product mango sorbet did not cause significant changes in the physiological responses such as blood pressure and heart rate, as well as parasympathetic nervous system activation (as determined by HF and LF/HF band HRV markers). It is also important to note that reduction of physiological responses via pharmacological interventions does not necessarily mean that the capacity to cope and manage stress is increased. Further food consumption studies with longer duration of consumption should be conducted to evaluate the use of L-THE as a supplement when consumed alongside other foods. It is anticipated that the results of this study will provide baseline information in understanding the activities of the human physiology and its effect on the stress response as well as the important notion to consider the effect food of matrixes have when constructing functional food ingredients.

Author Contributions: Conceptualization, J.W., A.J.M. and N.N.; Data curation, N.M.D.; Formal analysis, J.W., A.J.M. and E.N.G.; Investigation, J.W.; Methodology, D.S. and N.N.; Project administration, N.N.; Supervision, A.J.M. and N.N.; Writing—original draft, J.W.; Writing—review & editing, A.J.M., E.N.G., J.K., N.M.D., D.S., D.M. and N.N. All authors have read and agreed to the published version of the manuscript.

Funding: This project was funded by the University of Canberra Faculty of Health seed grant funding. J.W., is supported by an Australian Government Research Training Program scholarship. N.M.D. is supported by a Dementia Australia Research Foundation PhD scholarship. All other authors declare no funding sources.

Acknowledgments: This research was supported by the Faculty of Health Research Support Funding, University of Canberra, Canberra, ACT, Australia.

Conflicts of Interest: The authors declare no conflict of interest.

References

1. Kim, J.J.; Diamond, D.M. The stressed hippocampus, synaptic plasticity and lost memories. *Nat. Rev. Neurosci.* **2002**, *3*, 453–462. [CrossRef] [PubMed]
2. Russell, G.; Lightman, S. The human stress response. *Nat. Rev. Endocrinol.* **2019**, *15*, 525–534. [CrossRef] [PubMed]
3. Williams, J.L.; Everett, J.M.; D'Cunha, N.M.; Sergi, D.; Georgousopoulou, E.N.; Keegan, R.J.; McKune, A.J.; Mellor, D.D.; Anstice, N.; Naumovski, N. The Effects of Green Tea Amino Acid L-Theanine Consumption on the Ability to Manage Stress and Anxiety Levels: A Systematic Review. *Plant Foods Hum. Nutr.* **2019**, 1–12. [CrossRef] [PubMed]
4. Onakpoya, I.; Spencer, E.; Heneghan, C.; Thompson, M. The effect of green tea on blood pressure and lipid profile: A systematic review and meta-analysis of randomized clinical trials. *Nutr. Metab. Cardiovasc. Dis.* **2014**, *24*, 823–836. [CrossRef]
5. Lee, B.H.; Nam, T.G.; Park, N.Y.; Chun, O.K.; Koo, S.I.; Kim, D.-O. Estimated daily intake of phenolics and antioxidants from green tea consumption in the Korean diet. *Int. J. Food Sci. Nutr.* **2016**, *67*, 344–352. [CrossRef]
6. Williams, J.; Kellett, J.; Roach, P.D.; McKune, A.; Mellor, D.; Thomas, J.; Naumovski, N. L-Theanine as a Functional Food Additive: Its Role in Disease Prevention and Health Promotion. *Beverages* **2016**, *2*, 13. [CrossRef]
7. Naumovski, N.; Foscolou, A.; D'Cunha, N.M.; Tyrovolas, S.; Chrysohoou, C.; Sidossis, L.S.; Rallidis, L.; Matalas, A.-L.; Polychronopoulos, E.; Pitsavos, C.; et al. The Association between Green and Black Tea Consumption on Successful Aging: A Combined Analysis of the ATTICA and MEDiterranean ISlands (MEDIS) Epidemiological Studies. *Molecules* **2019**, *24*, 1862. [CrossRef]
8. Sergi, D.; Williams, L.M.; Thomas, J.; Mellor, D.D.; Naumovski, N. The effects of l-theanine and egcg on palmitic acid induced inflammation in mouse hypothalamic neuronal cell lines (mhypoe-n42). *JNIM* **2017**, *8*, 60–121. [CrossRef]
9. Vuong, Q.V.; Bowyer, M.C.; Roach, P.D. L-Theanine: Properties, synthesis and isolation from tea. *J. Sci. Food Agric.* **2011**, *91*, 1931–1939. [CrossRef] [PubMed]
10. Dodd, F.L.; Kennedy, D.O.; Riby, L.M.; Haskell-Ramsay, C.F. A double-blind, placebo-controlled study evaluating the effects of caffeine and L-theanine both alone and in combination on cerebral blood flow, cognition and mood. *Psychopharmacology* **2015**, *232*, 2563–2576. [CrossRef]
11. Naumovski, N.; Blades, B.L.; Roach, P.D. Food Inhibits the Oral Bioavailability of the Major Green Tea Antioxidant Epigallocatechin Gallate in Humans. *Antioxidants* **2015**, *4*, 373–393. [CrossRef] [PubMed]
12. Deka, A.; Vita, J.A. Tea and cardiovascular disease. *Pharmacol. Res.* **2011**, *64*, 136–145. [CrossRef] [PubMed]
13. Yoto, A.; Motoki, M.; Murao, S.; Yokogoshi, H. Effects of L-theanine or caffeine intake on changes in blood pressure under physical and psychological stresses. *J. Physiol. Anthropol.* **2012**, *31*, 28. [CrossRef] [PubMed]
14. Hidese, S.; Ogawa, S.; Ota, M.; Ishida, I.; Yasukawa, Z.; Ozeki, M.; Kunugi, H. Effects of L-Theanine Administration on Stress-Related Symptoms and Cognitive Functions in Healthy Adults: A Randomized Controlled Trial. *Nutrients* **2019**, *11*, 2362. [CrossRef]
15. Kimura, K.; Ozeki, M.; Juneja, L.R.; Ohira, H. L-Theanine reduces psychological and physiological stress responses. *Biol. Psychol.* **2007**, *74*, 39–45. [CrossRef]
16. McKune, A.J.; Bach, C.W.; Semple, S.J.; Dyer, B.J. Salivary cortisol and alpha-amylase responses to repeated bouts of downhill running. *Am. J. Hum. Biol.* **2014**, *26*, 850–855. [CrossRef]
17. Botek, M.; Krejci, J.; De Smet, S.; Gaba, A.; McKune, A.J. Heart rate variability and arterial oxygen saturation response during extreme normobaric hypoxia. *Auton. Neurosci.* **2015**, *190*, 40–45. [CrossRef]
18. Speer, K.E.; Semple, S.; Naumovski, N.; D'Cunha, N.M.; McKune, A.J. HPA axis function and diurnal cortisol in post-traumatic stress disorder: A systematic review. *Neurobiol. Stress* **2019**, *11*, 100180. [CrossRef]
19. Juneja, R.; Djong-Chi, C.; Tsutomu, O.; Yukiko, N.; Hidehiko, Y. L-theanine—A unique amino acid of green tea and its relaxation effect in humans. *Trends Food Sci. Tech.* **1999**, *10*, 199–204. [CrossRef]

20. Carroll, B.J. Use of the dexamethasone suppression test in depression. *J. Clin. Psychiatry* **1982**, *43*, 44–50.
21. Berntson, G.G.; Bigger, J.T., Jr.; Eckberg, D.L.; Grossman, P.; Kaufmann, P.G.; Malik, M.; Nagaraja, H.N.; Porges, S.W.; Saul, J.P.; Stone, P.H.; et al. Heart rate Variability: Origins, methods, and interpretive caveats. *Psychophysiology* **1997**, *34*, 623–648. [CrossRef] [PubMed]
22. Kim, H.-G.; Cheon, E.-J.; Bai, D.-S.; Lee, Y.H.; Koo, B.-H. Stress and Heart Rate Variability: A Meta-Analysis and Review of the Literature. *Psychiatry Investig.* **2018**, *15*, 235–245. [CrossRef] [PubMed]
23. Karatsoreos, I.N.; McEwen, B.S. Psychobiological allostasis: Resistance, resilience and vulnerability. *Trends Cogn. Sci.* **2011**, *15*, 576–584. [CrossRef]
24. Young, H.A.; Benton, D. Heart-rate variability: A biomarker to study the influence of nutrition on physiological and psychological health? *Behav. Pharmacol.* **2018**, *29*, 140–151. [CrossRef] [PubMed]
25. Forsyth, C.; Kouvari, M.; D'Cunha, N.M.; Georgousopoulou, E.N.; Panagiotakos, D.B.; Mellor, D.D.; Kellett, J.; Naumovski, N. The effects of the Mediterranean diet on rheumatoid arthritis prevention and treatment: A systematic review of human prospective studies. *Rheumatol. Int.* **2018**, *38*, 737–747. [CrossRef] [PubMed]
26. Zulfiqar, U.; Jurivich, D.A.; Gao, W.; Singer, D.H. Relation of high heart rate variability to healthy longevity. *Am. J. Cardiol.* **2010**, *105*, 1181–1185. [CrossRef] [PubMed]
27. Gottsater, A.; Ahlgren, A.R.; Taimour, S.; Sundkvist, G. Decreased heart rate variability may predict the progression of carotid atherosclerosis in type 2 diabetes. *Clin. Auton. Res.* **2006**, *16*, 228–234. [CrossRef]
28. Yoshioka, K.; Terasaki, J. Relationship between diabetic autonomic neuropathy and peripheral neuropathy as assessed by power spectral analysis of heart rate variations and vibratory perception thresholds. *Diabetes Res. Clin. Pract.* **1994**, *24*, 9–14. [CrossRef]
29. Scheid, L.; Ellinger, S.; Alteheld, B.; Herholz, H.; Ellinger, J.; Henn, T.; Helfrich, H.P.; Stehle, P. Kinetics of L-theanine uptake and metabolism in healthy participants are comparable after ingestion of L-theanine via capsules and green tea. *J. Nutr.* **2012**, *142*, 2091–2096. [CrossRef]
30. Williams, J.; Sergi, D.; McKune, A.J.; Georgousopoulou, E.N.; Mellor, D.D.; Naumovski, N. The beneficial health effects of green tea amino acid l-theanine in animal models: Promises and prospects for human trials. *Phytother. Res.* **2019**, *33*, 571–583. [CrossRef]
31. National Center for Biotechnology Information, United States National Library of Medicine. L-Theanine. Available online: http://pubchem.ncbi.nlm.nih.gov/compound/L-Theanine#section=Top (accessed on 18 November 2015).
32. Wing, L.M.; Reid, C.M.; Ryan, P.; Beilin, L.J.; Brown, M.A.; Jennings, G.L.; Johnston, C.I.; McNeil, J.J.; Marley, J.E.; Morgan, T.O.; et al. Second Australian National Blood Pressure Study (ANBP2). Australian Comparative Outcome Trial of ACE inhibitor- and diuretic-based treatment of hypertension in the elderly. Management Committee on Behalf of the High Blood Pressure Research Council of Australia. *Clin. Exp. Hypertens.* **1997**, *19*, 779–791. [CrossRef] [PubMed]
33. Sookan, T.; McKune, A.J. Heart rate variability in physically active individuals: Reliability and gender characteristics. *Cardiovasc. J. Afr.* **2012**, *23*, 67–72. [CrossRef] [PubMed]
34. Potter, J.F.; Heseltine, D.; Hartley, G.; Matthews, J.; Macdonald, I.A.; James, O.F.W. Effects of Meal Composition on the Postprandial Blood Pressure, Catecholamine and Insulin Changes in Elderly Subjects. *Clin. Sci.* **1989**, *77*, 265–272. [CrossRef] [PubMed]
35. Van der Pijl, P.C.; Chen, L.; Mulder, T.P. Human disposition of L-theanine in tea or aqueous solution. *J. Funct. Foods* **2010**, *2*, 239–244. [CrossRef]
36. Giesbrecht, T.; Rycroft, J.A.; Rowson, M.J.; De Bruin, E.A. The combination of L-theanine and caffeine improves cognitive performance and increases subjective alertness. *Nutr. Neurosci.* **2010**, *13*, 283–290. [CrossRef]
37. Rogers, P.J.; Smith, J.E.; Heatherley, S.V.; Pleydell-Pearce, C.W. Time for tea: Mood, blood pressure and cognitive performance effects of caffeine and theanine administered alone and together. *Psychopharmacology* **2008**, *195*, 569–577. [CrossRef]
38. White, D.J.; de Klerk, S.; Woods, W.; Gondalia, S.; Noonan, C.; Scholey, A.B. Anti-Stress, Behavioural and Magnetoencephalography Effects of an l-Theanine-Based Nutrient Drink: A Randomised, Double-Blind, Placebo-Controlled, Crossover Trial. *Nutrients* **2016**, *8*, 53. [CrossRef]
39. Montopoli, M.; Stevens, L.; Smith, C.J.; Montopoli, G.; Passino, S.; Brown, S.; Camou, L.; Carson, K.; Maaske, S.; Knights, K.; et al. The Acute Electrocortical and Blood Pressure Effects of Chocolate. *Neuro Regul.* **2015**, *2*, 3–28. [CrossRef]

40. Kakuda, T.; Nozawa, A.; Sugimoto, A.; Niino, H. Inhibition by theanine of binding of [3H]AMPA, [3H]kainate, and [3H]MDL 105,519 to glutamate receptors. *Biosci. Biotechnol. Biochem.* **2002**, *66*, 2683–2686. [CrossRef]
41. Unno, K.; Tanida, N.; Ishii, N.; Yamamoto, H.; Iguchi, K.; Hoshino, M.; Takeda, A.; Ozawa, H.; Ohkubo, T.; Juneja, L.R.; et al. Anti-stress effect of theanine on students during pharmacy practice: Positive correlation among salivary alpha-amylase activity, trait anxiety and subjective stress. *Pharmacol. Biochem. Behav.* **2013**, *111*, 128–135. [CrossRef]
42. Yoneda, Y.; Kawada, K.; Kuramoto, N. Selective Upregulation by Theanine of Slc38a1 Expression in Neural Stem Cell for Brain Wellness. *Molecules* **2020**, *25*, 347. [CrossRef] [PubMed]
43. Unno, K.; Sumiyoshi, A.; Konishi, T.; Hayashi, M.; Taguchi, K.; Muguruma, Y.; Inoue, K.; Iguchi, K.; Nonaka, H.; Kawashima, R.; et al. Theanine, the Main Amino Acid in Tea, Prevents Stress-Induced Brain Atrophy by Modifying Early Stress Responses. *Nutrients* **2020**, *12*, 174. [CrossRef] [PubMed]
44. Kakuda, T.; Hinoi, E.; Abe, A.; Nozawa, A.; Ogura, M.; Yoneda, Y. Theanine, an ingredient of green tea, inhibits [3H]glutamine transport in neurons and astroglia in rat brain. *J. Neurosci. Res.* **2008**, *86*, 1846–1856. [CrossRef] [PubMed]
45. Yokogoshi, H.; Kato, Y.; Sagesaka, Y.M.; Takihara-Matsuura, T.; Kakuda, T.; Takeuchi, N. Reduction Effect of Theanine on Blood Pressure and Brain 5-Hydroxyindoles in Spontaneously Hypertensive Rats. *Biosci. Biotech. Biochem.* **1995**, *59*, 615–618. [CrossRef] [PubMed]
46. Yokogoshi, H.; Kobayashi, M.; Mochizuki, M.; Terashima, T. Effect of theanine, r-glutamylethylamide, on brain monoamines and striatal dopamine release in conscious rats. *Neurochem. Res.* **1998**, *23*, 667–673. [CrossRef] [PubMed]

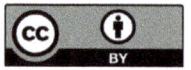

© 2020 by the authors. Licensee MDPI, Basel, Switzerland. This article is an open access article distributed under the terms and conditions of the Creative Commons Attribution (CC BY) license (http://creativecommons.org/licenses/by/4.0/).

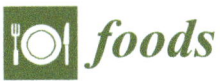

Article

Long-Chain Polyunsaturated Fatty Acids Are Associated with Blood Pressure and Hypertension over 10-Years in Black South African Adults Undergoing Nutritional Transition

Manja M. Zec [1,2,*], Aletta E. Schutte [3,4], Cristian Ricci [1], Jeannine Baumgartner [1], Iolanthe M. Kruger [5] and Cornelius M. Smuts [1]

1. Centre of Excellence for Nutrition, North-West University, 2520 Potchefstroom, South Africa
2. Centre of Excellence in Nutrition and Metabolism, Institute for Medical Research, University of Belgrade, 11000 Belgrade, Serbia
3. Hypertension in Africa Research Team (HART), North-West University, 2520 Potchefstroom, South Africa
4. Medical Research Council Unit: Hypertension and Cardiovascular Disease, North-West University, 2520 Potchefstroom, South Africa
5. Africa Unit for Transdisciplinary Health Research (AUTHeR), North-West University, 2520 Potchefstroom, South Africa
* Correspondence: manjazec@gmail.com; Tel.: +27-18-299-2086

Received: 16 August 2019; Accepted: 2 September 2019; Published: 6 September 2019

Abstract: Nutritional transition in Africa is linked with increased blood pressure (BP). We examined 10-year fatty acid status and longitudinal associations between individual long-chain polyunsaturated fatty acids (PUFA), BP and status of hypertension (≥140/90 mmHg and/or medication use) in black South Africans. We included 300 adults (>30 years) participating in the Prospective Urban Rural Epidemiology study, and analysed data from three consecutive examinations (2005, 2010 and 2015 study years). Fatty acids in plasma phospholipids were analysed by gas chromatography-mass spectrometry. We applied sequential linear mixed models for continuous outcomes and generalized mixed models for the hypertension outcome, in the complete sample and separately in urban and rural subjects. Mean baseline systolic/diastolic BP was 137/89 mmHg. Ten-year hypertension status increased among rural (48.6% to 68.6%, $p = 0.001$) and tended to decrease among urban subjects (67.5% to 61.9%, $p = 0.253$). Regardless of urbanisation, n-6 PUFA increased and eicosapentaenoic acid (EPA, C20:5 n-3) decreased over the 10-years. Subjects in the highest tertile of arachidonic acid (C20:4 n-6) had 3.81 mmHg lower systolic (95% confidence interval (CI): −7.07, −0.54) and 3.82 mmHg lower diastolic BP (DBP) (95% CI: −5.70, −1.95) compared to the reference tertile, irrespective of lifestyle and clinical confounders. Similarly, osbond acid (C22:5 n-6) was inversely associated with DBP. Over the 10-years, subjects in the highest EPA tertile presented with +2.92 and +1.94 mmHg higher SBP and DBP, respectively, and with 1.46 higher odds of being hypertensive. In black South African adults, individual plasma n-6 PUFA were inversely associated with BP, whereas EPA was adversely associated with hypertension, supporting implementation of dietary fat quality in national cardiovascular primary prevention strategies.

Keywords: black Africans; blood pressure; hypertension; long-chain polyunsaturated fatty acids; longitudinal study; nutritional transition; PUFA

1. Introduction

Urbanisation in sub-Saharan Africa followed by increased consumption of energy-dense food [1], is linked with an increase in cardiovascular disease, obesity and diabetes [2], and the highest prevalence of mean blood pressure (BP) since 1980 [3]. Among black South African adults (>30 years) participating in a large-scale Prospective Urban Rural Epidemiology (PURE) study, a five-year increase in hypertension rate has been reported [4]. Nutritional interventions remain a cost-effective approach in suppressing the hypertension burden in the population. Baseline data from the PURE study indicate low total fat and omega-3 (n-3) intake in black South Africans [5]. In the same study, dietary n-3 long-chain polyunsaturated fatty acids (PUFA) were associated with serum lipids. Dietary eicosapentaenoic acid (EPA; C20:5 n-3) was associated with dyslipidemia and docosahexaenoic acid (DHA; C22:6 n-3) with favourable lipid status in the population [5]. These results indicate a unique metabolic profile in black South Africans related to fat catabolism and a specific role of individual fatty acids in cardiometabolic function.

Long-chain n-3 PUFA from marine foods demonstrate BP-lowering effects [6]. Clinical studies show that long-chain n-3 PUFA consumption diminishes the risk of cardiac death, potentially through regulation of triglycerides, heart rate and BP [7]. Measurement of the intake remains a challenge, since questionnaires are imprecise in differentiating intake of individual long-chain fatty acids. Self-reported information from dietary questionnaires is further limited by recall bias and participants' non-compliance to fat-intake related questions [8]. Fatty acids in plasma phospholipids are however reliable biomarkers reflecting fat intake of the preceding 6-8 weeks [9]. Dietary fatty acids are endogenously catalysed by desaturase-5 and desaturase-6 enzymes encoded by FADS1 and FADS2 genes, respectively. The conversion results in the formation of long-chain PUFA with diverse physiological functions. Plasma fatty acids are of raising importance as prognostic biomarkers of cardiovascular disease [10]. Data from the Women's Health Initiative study show inverse association between n-3 group and coronary heart disease risk in post-menopausal women [11]. A recent review underlined the importance of individual circulating fatty acids with regards to total and cause-specific mortality, type 2 diabetes mellitus and cardiometabolic indices [10]. Plasma fatty acids have been associated with BP [12–14], and observational data suggest protective associations of individual circulating n-3 long-chain PUFA with BP [15,16]. In middle-aged and elderly Chinese community dwellers, serum patterns presenting with high DHA levels were inversely associated with BP [12] and hypertension status [17]. Recent data from the PURE study showed association between plasma phospholipid fatty acid patterns and obesity and metabolic syndrome in black South African adults [18], however the link with vascular function has not yet been examined in the population.

Therefore, the objective of this longitudinal study was to evaluate the relationship between fat intake and BP in black South Africans. We measured and reported fatty acids in plasma phospholipids over 10 years, in a sample of black South Africans participating in the PURE and residing in rapidly urbanizing areas. To address the study objective, we examined the associations between individual long-chain n-3 and n-6 PUFA with BP and hypertension status over the 10-years. We also evaluated the 10-year associations separately in subjects residing in urban and rural areas.

2. Materials and Methods

2.1. Study Design and Selection of Study Sample

This study formed part of the South African cohort of the PURE study, an international study investigating health implications linked with urbanisation in low-, middle- and high-income countries [19]. The cohort included 2010 (1260 women and 750 men at baseline) randomly selected black adults (>30 years), from urban and rural areas of the North West Province, without use of chronic medication and/or any self-reported acute illness. Permission for the study was obtained from the provincial Department of Health. Trained fieldworkers fluent in both English and Setswana conveyed all information. All subjects voluntarily gave written informed consent for the participation in 2005, continuous consent throughout the study and again in 2010 and 2015. The study protocol adhered to the 1983 Declaration of Helsinki and was approved by the Health Research Ethics Committee of the Faculty of Health Sciences at the North-West University (Potchefstroom campus). Privacy and confidentiality were ensured during the data-gathering process, data and sample storage and management.

For the purposes of this study and analysis we applied a repeated-measures design and included data and assessments from 2005 (baseline), 2010 and 2015 (follow-up). A sub-cohort of 711 subjects were randomly selected at 2010 (Supplementary Materials Figure S1) and fatty acid analysed accordingly. Due to the loss to follow-up in the 2015 study year, we ended up with 300 complete sets of samples across the 3 study years, inclusive of fatty acid profiles and vascular outcomes. The 300 corresponding subjects were thus included in the longitudinal analysis.

2.2. Clinical and Biological Measurements

Fasting blood samples were collected from the antecubital vein with a sterile winged infusion set and were with minimal stasis. The samples were collected by a registered nurse and stored at $-80\,^\circ$C. In rural areas the samples were stored at $-18\,^\circ$C up to 5 days; afterwards transported to the laboratory facility and stored at $-80\,^\circ$C until analysis. Plasma phospholipid fatty acid composition was analysed as described previously [20]. Briefly, lipids were extracted with chloroform: methanol (2:1 v/v) from thawed ethylenediaminetetraacetic acid-plasma samples according to the modified Folch method [21]. The phospholipid fatty acid fractions were subsequently isolated by thin layer chromatography, further transmethylated to fatty acid methyl esters, and analysed by quadrupole gas chromatography electron ionization mass spectrometry using an Agilent Technologies 7890 A GC system [20]. Levels of each individual fatty acid were expressed as a percentage of the total phospholipid fatty acid pool in plasma. To examine longitudinal associations with vascular function, we used data for the long-chain n-3 fatty acids: EPA, DHA and docosapentaenoic acid (C22:5 n-3); and n-6 fatty acids: dihomo-γ-linolenic acid (DGLA, C20:4 n-6), arachidonic acid (AA, C20:4 n-6), adrenic acid (C22:4 n-6), and docosapentaenoic acid (osbond acid, C22:5 n-6).

Brachial BP was measured in duplicate in a sitting position by using a validated OMRON device (Omron Healthcare, Kyoto, Japan) after subjects rested for 10 min, as reported elsewhere [4]. To be categorized as hypertensive, the participants had to exceed either SBP (140) or DBP (90) or both thresholds (or had to use antihypertensive medication) [22]. The PURE-standardized demographic, socio-economic and lifestyle questionnaires were interviewer administered [19]. Education was confirmed if any formal education was present. Quantitative FFQ and the physical activity index questionnaire previously developed and validated for South Africans were used [23,24]. The FFQ was conducted in the morning on the study visit day. Study participants were provided with a list of food items (food or drinks) and were asked how often they had consumed specific foods or drinks on average in the preceding year. Assessment of height, weight, waist circumference, serum lipids and other biochemical measurements were described previously [4,5].

2.3. Statistical Analyses

Statistical analysis was performed using SAS 9.4 (SAS Institute Inc, Cary, NC, USA). Continuous variables were checked for the distribution by visual inspection of histogram and skewness. Normal, non-normal and categorical data are presented as mean $\pm$ SD, median [25th, 75th percentile] and percentages, respectively. Baseline between-subject differences across urbanisation areas were tested by independent t-test and Mann Whitney test, for normal and non-normal data, respectively. Between-subject differences across the three study years were analysed by general linear model. Pearson's correlation coefficients were computed to evaluate the relationship between plasma long-chain phospholipid PUFA, n-3 intake (cumulative intake of dietary α-linolenic acid (ALA, C18:3 n-3), EPA and DHA) and marine fatty acid intake (cumulative intake of EPA and DHA).

We evaluated 10-year associations between individual n-3 and n-6 long-chain PUFA (exposures) and the outcomes, by inclusion of data for the three study points. We applied linear mixed models for continuous outcomes (SBP and DBP) and generalized mixed models for the outcome of hypertension, with individual exposure fatty acids included as tertiles of the plasma phospholipid content. Sequential regression-based models were applied: Model 1 with fatty acid predictors controlled for age, gender and level of urbanisation (urban or rural); Model 2 further controlled for lifestyle confounders, including level of education (no education or any kind of formal education), self-reported use of tobacco (current, former or never used), use of hypertension medication (yes or no), body mass index, physical activity index and dietary intake of alcohol (g per day). The urbanisation status was treated as random factor, and repeated measures design was accounted for by use of adequate syntax within the procedures. We performed a prespecified subgroup analysis, stratified by urbanisation status (rural and urban areas). The level of significance was set at 0.05 (2-tailed).

2.4. Sensitivity Analyses

We further tested whether multivariable-adjusted associations were independent on dietary and fat intake in three consecutive steps: adjusting for total energy intake, following total fat and carbohydrate intake, and lastly ratio of monounsaturated to saturated fat intake, and soluble fiber intake, latter known to be protective towards vascular health [25,26]. We also tested whether our associations survived upon adjustment for potential effect mediators linked with BP, including total cholesterol, triglycerides, fasting glucose, and γ-glutamyl transferase reported to be associated with hypertension in this population [4].

3. Results

3.1. Baseline Characteristics of the 300 Rural and Urban Black South Africans

The study sample included 300 black South Africans (mean age = 53.12 ± 9.83), out of which 91 were men, 140 rural residents (46.7%), and 42.3% overweight subjects, mostly women (53.6% and 16.5% women and men who are overweight, respectively, $p < 0.0001$). In total, 19.7% and 23% subjects had elevated total cholesterol and triglycerides, respectively. Only 2.3% of participants were either diagnosed with type 2 diabetes or actively taking anti-diabetic medications.

Urban subjects presented with higher hypertension prevalence and had higher SBP and DBP, then rural residents. The intake of total energy, total carbohydrates, total fat, and specific fat groups were higher among urban subjects (Table 1).

Table 1. Baseline characteristics of the 300 rural and urban black South Africans.

	Complete Sample (n 300)	Rural Areas (n 140)	Urban Areas (n 160)	p-Value [1]
Gender, men, n (%)	91 (30.33)	39 (27.86)	52 (32.5)	0.385
Any education, n (%)	190 (64.63)	65 (47.10)	125 (80.13)	<0.001
Current smokers, n (%)	155 (51.84)	74 (52.86)	81 (50.94)	0.201
Former smokers, n (%)	135 (45.15)	59 (42.14)	76 (47.8)	
Clinical parameters				
Age, years	53.12 (9.83)	52.20 (9.16)	53.93 (10.34)	0.130
Body mass index, kg m^{-2}	23.91 [19.93, 29.61]	23.39 [19.44, 29.43]	24.03 [20.43, 29.61]	0.172
Waist circumference. cm	80.68 (12.99)	79.84 (13.43)	81.42 (12.60)	0.295
Systolic blood pressure, mmHg	136.54 (3.29)	131.56 (22.81)	140.91 (22.89)	0.001
Diastolic blood pressure, mmHg	89.04 (12.69)	87.10 (13.33)	90.75 (11.87)	0.013
Fasting glucose, mmol L^{-1}	5.11 (1.53)	4.87 (1.08)	5.32 (1.82)	0.010
Total cholesterol, mmol L^{-1}	5.22 (1.30)	5.12 (1.32)	5.31 (1.27)	0.193
HDL-c, mmol L^{-1}	1.58 (0.64)	1.55 (0.65)	1.62 (0.64)	0.338
LDL-c, mmol L^{-1}	3.01 (1.18)	3.00 (1.16)	3.03 (1.19)	0.820
Tryglicerides, mmol L^{-1}	1.15 [0.84, 1.68]	1.10 [0.84, 1.53]	1.23 [0.84, 1.75]	0.142
Weighted physical activity index	2.76 [2.49, 3.17]	3.07 [2.61, 3.43]	2.62 [2.38, 2.89]	<0.0001
GGT, U L^{-1}	43.00 [29.00, 85.06]	37.30 [26.90, 64.35]	50.29 [34.38, 95.50]	0.001
hsCRP, mg L^{-1}	3.19 [1.04, 7.52]	3.32 [0.90, 7.36]	2.90 [1.07, 8.39]	0.722
Use of hypertension medication, n (%)	55 (18.3)	27 (19.3)	28 (17.5)	0.691
Hypertensive, n (%)	176 (58.7)	68 (48.6)	108 (67.5)	<0.001

Table 1. Cont.

	Complete Sample (n 300)	Rural Areas (n 140)	Urban Areas (n 160)	p-Value [1]
		Dietary intake		
Energy, kJ	7251.15 [5259.26, 9689.23]	6103.36 [4681.22, 7928.72]	8453.99 [5824.48, 11439.46]	<0.0001
Total fat, g	43.14 [27.73, 63.05]	30.53 [21.94, 42.22]	59.04 [40.89, 82.64]	<0.0001
Saturated fat, g	9.97 [5.98, 16.29]	6.61 [3.88, 9.20]	15.18 [10.10, 21.39]	<0.0001
Monounsaturated fat, g	10.92 [6.10, 18.05]	6.79 [4.20, 10.00]	16.20 [11.14, 24.69]	<0.0001
Polyunsaturated fat, g	13.55 [7.85, 20.23]	9.59 [6.50, 14.26]	17.10 [11.49, 23.60]	<0.0001
n-3 intake, mg	314.10 [188.98, 476.17]	209.19 [137.58, 314.34]	425.59 [298.12, 608.72]	<0.0001
EPA+DHA intake, mg	109.91 [49.20, 199.49]	79.91 [34.66, 137.56]	130.48 [58.90, 230.20]	<0.0001
Total carbohydrate, g	279.98 (129.89)	256.77 (113.15)	300.29 (140.15)	0.003
Total fibre, g	21.35 (10.48)	18.62 (8.11)	23.75 (11.68)	<0.0001
Soluble fibre, g	1.40 [0.84, 2.32]	0.97 [0.66, 1.43]	2.12 [1.28, 3.32]	<0.0001
Alcohol, g	0.00 [0.00, 11.50]	0.00 [0.00, 5.71]	0.10 [0.00, 15.33]	0.010

HDL-c, High-density lipoprotein cholesterol; LDL-c, Low-density lipoprotein cholesterol; GGT, γ-glutamyl transferase; EPA, Eicosapentaenoic acid; DHA, Docosahexaenoic acid; n-3, Intake of EPA, DHA and plant-originated α-linolenic acid. Data are presented as mean (SD), median [25th, 75th] or percentage for categorical variables.
[1] Significance values calculated by use of independent t-test or Mann-Whitney test.

3.2. Ten-Year Changes in Blood Pressure and Status of Hypertension

Within all 300 subjects, we observed a non-significant increase in hypertension rate (58.7%, 61.3% and 65% in 2005, 2010 and 2015, respectively; $p = 0.210$). There was a significant increase in the hypertension rate in rural residents (48.6%, 51.4% and 68.6% in 2005, 2010 and 2015, respectively; $p = 0.001$), and a non-significant decrease within urban dwellers (67.5%, 70% and 61.9% in 2005, 2010 and 2015, respectively; $p = 0.253$). At baseline and in 2010 there were significantly more hypertensive subjects in urban areas, with no differences in 2015. SBP and DBP significantly decreased across the 10-years in urban areas (Supplementary Materials Table S1).

3.3. Ten-Year Changes in Long-Chain Plasma Phospholipid Fatty Acids

There was a significant decrease in γ-linolenic acid. Long-chain n-6 PUFA (DGLA, AA, adrenic and osbond acid) increased and long-chain n-3 (EPA and DHA) decreased across the 10 years (Table 2). Ten-year fatty acid status across urbanisation areas is presented in Supplementary Materials Table S2. Regardless of urbanisation level, we observed increases in DGLA, AA and osbond acid. In urbans only, adrenic acid increased and EPA and DHA decreased over the 10-years. In rural subjects, docosapentaenoic acid and DHA content increased and EPA tended to decrease.

Table 2. Plasma phospholipid fatty acid status across 10 years in 300 black South Africans.

	Study Year			p [1]
	2005	2010	2015	
Myristic acid, 14:0	0.27 (0.01)	0.27 (0.01)	0.33 (0.03)	<0.0001
Palmitic acid, 16:0	26.93 (0.31)	27.17 (0.45)	24.79 (0.64)	<0.0001
Palmitoleic acid, 16:1 n-7	0.86 [0.76, 0.96]	0.83 [0.70, 0.91]	0.93 [0.79, 1.04]	0.086
Stearic acid, 18:0	15.26 (0.96)	14.92 (0.61)	14.19 (0.07)	<0.0001
Oleic acid, 18:1 n-9	8.84 [8.35, 9.27]	8.48 [7.88, 8.95]	8.33 [7.73, 8.63]	0.025
Mead, 20:3 n-9	0.25 [0.25, 0.26]	0.24 [0.22, 0.25]	0.27 [0.19, 0.28]	0.216
Linoleic acid, 18:2 n-6	16.03 (0.41)	16.70 (1.01)	16.07 (0.28)	0.579
γ-Linolenic, 18:3 n-6	0.12 [0.11, 0.12]	0.12 [0.11, 0.13]	0.11 [0.10, 0.11]	0.018
Dihomo-γ-linolenic, 20:3 n-6	2.91 (0.09)	2.89 (0.08)	3.48 (0.19)	<0.0001
Arachidonic acid, 20:4 n-6	13.57 (0.24)	14.65 (0.31)	18.13 (0.37)	<0.0001
Adrenic, 22:4 n-6	0.60 (0.07)	0.70 (0.01)	0.66 (0.02)	<0.0001
Osbond, 22:5 n-6	0.57 [0.56, 0.67]	0.72 [0.70, 0.73]	1.07 [0.93, 1.09]	<0.0001
α-linolenic acid, 18:3 n-3	0.09 [0.09, 0.09]	0.09 [0.09, 0.11]	0.07 [0.07, 0.08]	<0.0001
EPA, 20:5 n-3	0.78 [0.59, 0.80]	0.47 [0.45, 0.60]	0.55 [0.52, 0.59]	<0.0001
Docosapentaenoic, 22:5 n-3	1.41 (0.02)	1.42 (0.19)	1.53 (0.09)	0.001
DHA, 22:6 n-3	4.56 (0.61)	3.88 (0.11)	4.33 (0.14)	0.009

EPA, Eicosapentaenoic acid; DHA, Docosahexaenoic acid. Age and urbanization factor-adjusted data presented as mean (SD) or median [25th, 75th]. [1] Probability trends associated with changes over 10-years calculated by general linear model adjusted for age and urbanization factor.

3.4. Relationship Between Dietary Intake of N-3 Fatty Acids and Long-Chain Fatty Acids in Plasma Phospholipids

A HeatMap of Pearson correlations among baseline intake of *n*-3 fatty acids and long-chain plasma phospholipid fatty acids is presented in Figure 1.

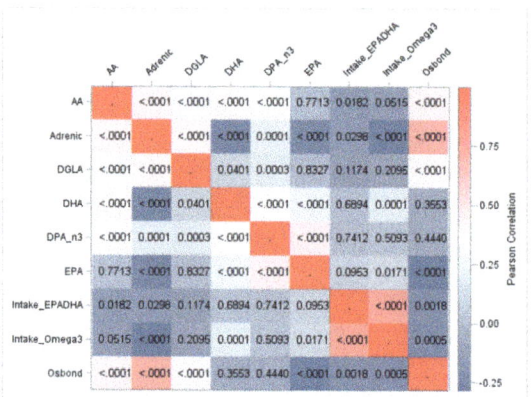

Figure 1. Baseline correlations between intake of *n*-3 fats and long-chain plasma fatty acids in 300 black South Africans: HeatMap of Pearson coefficients. DGLA, dihomo-γ-linoleic acid; AA, arachidonic acid; EPA, Eicosapentaenoic acid; DPA_n3, docosapentaenoic acid; DHA, Docosahexaenoic acid; Intake_EPADHA, Cumulative intake of preformed EPA and DHA; Intake_Omega3, Cumulative intake of EPA, DHA and plant-originated essential α-linolenic acid; <.0001, denotes statistical threshold (p) of < 0.0001 associated with correlation pair.

Cumulative *n*-3 intake was correlated with status of EPA and DHA, and negatively correlated with *n*-6 long-chain PUFA: AA ($r = -0.113$, $p = 0.052$), adrenic acid ($r = -0.280$, $p = < 0.0001$) and osbond acid ($r = -0.198$, $p = 0.001$) (Supplementary Materials Table S3). Cumulative intake of preformed EPA and DHA did not correlate with status of any long-chain *n*-3 PUFA, yet negatively correlated with long-chain *n*-6 PUFA: AA ($r = -0.136$, $p = 0.018$), adrenic acid ($r = -0.126$, $p = 0.030$) and osbond acid ($r = -0.180$, $p = 0.002$).

Fatty acids in plasma phospholipids within either the *n*-3 or *n*-6 group were correlated among each other. Adrenic acid inversely correlated with EPA and DHA. Osbond acid inversely correlated with EPA, while the inverse relationship with DPA and DHA did not reach statistical significance (Supplementary Materials Table S3).

3.5. Ten-Year Associations between Long-Chain Plasma Phospholipid Fatty Acids with Blood Pressure and Hypertension in Black South African Adults

3.5.1. Associations between N-3 Long-Chain Fatty Acids and Blood Pressure

Subjects in the highest tertile of plasma EPA content over the 10-years had 1.94 mmHg higher DBP in comparison with subjects in the lowest (multivariable β for T3 vs. T1: 1.94 (95% CI: 0.01, 3.87)), regardless of age, gender, BMI, educational background, intake of alcohol, smoking status, level of physical activity and use of hypertension medication (Table 3).

Urban subjects within the highest EPA content were with higher SBP (Supplementary Materials Table S4). DHA was inversely associated with DBP in rural dwellers (multivariable β for T3 vs. T1: −3.91 (95% CI: −7.04, −0.78).

Table 3. Ten-year associations between plasma phospholipid long-chain fatty acids and blood pressure in 300 black South Africans.

	Systolic Blood Pressure		Diastolic Blood Pressure	
	β (95% CI)	p^3	β (95% CI)	p^3
Long-chain *n*-3 fatty acids				
EPA, 20:5 *n*-3				
T1	ref.		ref.	
T2 [1]	1.89 (−1.40, 5.18)	0.322	1.44 (−0.44, 3.32)	0.143
T3	2.41 (−0.89, 5.70)		1.80 (−0.09, 3.69)	
T2 [2]	2.39 (−0.95, 5.72)	0.191	1.37 (−0.56, 3.30)	0.132
T3	2.92 (−0.41, 6.26)		1.94 (0.01, 3.87)	
Docosapentaenoic, 22:5 *n*-3				
T1	ref.		ref.	
T2 [1]	0.91 (−2.39, 4.22)	0.284	0.58 (−1.31, 2.48)	0.056
T3	−1.75 (−5.26, 1.75)		−1.69 (−3.69, 0.30)	
T2 [2]	0.22 (−3.10, 3.53)	0.349	0.33 (−1.59, 2.24)	0.068
T3	−2.11 (−5.63, 1.41)		−1.86 (−3.88, 0.17)	
DHA, 22:6 *n*-3				
T1	ref.		ref.	
T2 [1]	−0.92 (−4.31, 2.47)	0.386	−0.76 (−2.70, 1.18)	0.275
T3	−2.48 (−6.08, 1.11)		−1.68 (−3.73, 0.38)	
T2 [2]	−0.37 (−3.79, 3.06)	0.427	−0.51 (−2.49, 1.46)	0.358
T3	−2.21 (−5.86, 1.44)		−1.50 (−3.60, 0.60)	
Long-chain *n*-6 fatty acids				
Dihomo-γ-linolenic acid, 20:3 *n*-6				
T1	ref.		ref.	
T2 [1]	1.40 (−1.93, 4.73)	0.419	0.55 (−1.36, 2.46)	0.396
T3	−0.77 (−4.17, 2.63)		−0.75 (−2.70, 1.19)	
T2 [2]	0.68 (−2.70, 4.06)	0.392	0.23 (−1.72, 2.19)	0.305
T3	−1.59 (−5.07, 1.89)		−1.19 (−3.20, 0.82)	
Arachidonic acid, 20:4 *n*-6				
T1	ref.		ref.	
T2 [1]	−0.06 (−3.29, 3.16)	0.048	−0.83 (−2.66, 1.00)	<0.0001
T3	−3.50 (−6.73, −0.27)		−3.76 (−5.59, −1.93)	
T2 [2]	0.17 (−3.06, 3.39)	0.024	−0.62 (−2.47, 1.22)	<0.0001
T3	−3.81 (−7.07, −0.54)		−3.82 (−5.70, −1.95)	
Adrenic acid, 22:4 *n*-6				
T1	ref.		ref.	
T2 [1]	−1.87 (−5.11, 1.37)	0.327	0.03 (−1.83, 1.88)	0.999
T3	0.45 (−3.02, 3.92)		−0.02 (−2.00, 1.97)	
T2 [2]	−2.56 (−5.79, 0.68)	0.195	−0.23 (−2.10, 1.65)	0.943
T3	0.00 (−3.52, 3.53)		0.09 (−1.94, 2.13)	
Osbond acid, 22:5 *n*-6				
T1	ref.		ref.	
T2 [1]	−1.74 (−4.97, 1.48)	0.449	−1.22 (−3.05, 0.61)	0.002
T3	−2.03 (−5.51, 1.45)		−3.47 (−5.44, −1.49)	
T2 [2]	−1.96 (−5.18, 1.26)	0.197	−1.22 (−3.07, 0.63)	0.001
T3	−3.20 (−6.73, 0.33)		−3.71 (−5.73, −1.70)	

EPA, Eicosapentaenoic acid; DHA, Docosahexaenoic acid; T1, T2, T3, Increasing tertiles of plasma phospholipid fatty acid content. [1] Model 1 adjusted for age, gender and urbanization factor. [2] Model 2 further adjusted for level of education, use of tobacco, use of hypertension medication, body mass index, physical activity index and dietary intake of alcohol (g). [3] Probability values associated with β estimating absolute change in blood pressure (in mmHg) with regards to 10-year change in a fatty acid level.

3.5.2. Associations between N-6 Long-Chain Fatty Acids and Blood Pressure

Across the 10 years AA was inversely associated with SBP and DBP (Table 3). Subjects in the highest tertile were with 3.81 and 3.82 mmHg lower SBP and DBP, respectively, in comparison with subjects within the reference tertile (multivariable β for T3 vs. T1: −3.81 (95% CI: −7.07, −0.54) for SBP and −3.82 (95% CI: −5.70, −1.95) for DBP). Osbond acid was inversely associated with DBP (Table 3). Subjects in the highest tertile had 3.71 mmHg lower DBP in comparison with reference tertile (multivariable β for T3 vs. T1: −3.71 (95% CI: −5.73, −1.70)).

The inverse associations remained significant in urban residents for both AA and osbond acid, and osbond acid was also inversely associated with SBP (Supplementary Materials Table S4). In urban dwellers DGLA was inversely associated with DBP.

3.5.3. Associations between Long-Chain Plasma Fatty Acids and Status of Hypertension

Plasma phospholipid fatty acids were not associated with 10-years status of hypertension in the 300 black South African adults, except for EPA (Figure 2). Subjects in the highest tertile of EPA content were with 1.46 higher odds of being hypertensive across the 10-years, in comparison with those in the reference tertile (multivariable OR for T3 vs. T1: 1.46 (95% CI: 1.03, 2.08)) (Supplementary Materials Table S5). Adverse relationship of DGLA was lost upon controlling for potential confounders.

EPA remained adversely associated with 10-year hypertension status only in rural subjects within the highest tertile of the content. Furthermore, DGLA and osbond acid were adversely associated upon controlling for confounders known to influence the status. No associations were seen among urban dwellers.

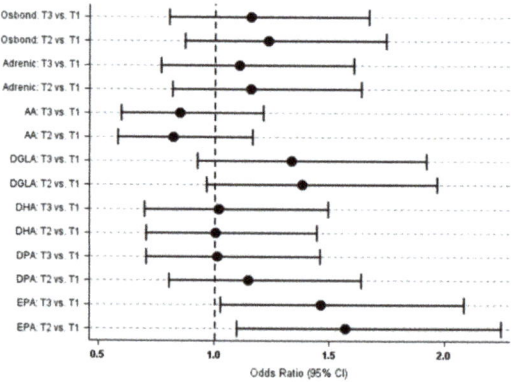

Figure 2. Multivariable odds ratio of being hypertensive across 10-years depending on the individual fatty acid content in plasma phospholipids in 300 black South Africans. AA, Arachidonic acid; DGLA, Dihomo-γ-linolenic acid, EPA, Eicosapentaenoic acid; DPA, docosapentaenoic acid; DHA, Docosahexaenoic acid; T1, T2, T3, Increasing tertiles of each plasma phospholipid fatty acid content.

3.5.4. Sensitivity Analyses

Observed 10-year associations with BP and hypertension status remained consistent upon sensitivity analyses evaluating contribution of dietary intake affecting fat metabolism, and serum biomarkers.

4. Discussion

Our study showed that in black middle-aged and elderly South Africans living in rapidly urbanizing areas, individual long-chain plasma phospholipid PUFA were associated with BP across 10 years. The n-6 fatty acids were protectively associated with office SBP and DBP, while subjects with the highest EPA content presented with higher DBP. The relationships were independent of age, gender, BMI, educational background, intake of alcohol, smoking status, level of physical activity, use of hypertension medication, total energy and intake of fat, and glucolipid biomarkers. Observed relationships between individual PUFA and vascular health confer the role of dietary fat quality in tailoring population-specific nutritional policies in black South Africans.

In our study EPA was adversely associated with 10-years status of hypertension. Previous studies suggest favourable associations of EPA intake with vascular function [7,27,28] and cardiovascular events [29]. In a prospective study among 1477 adult community dwellers, subjects in the highest quartile of erythrocyte EPA content had significantly lower SBP and DBP across 3 years [30]. However, the latter study included fatty acid biomarkers measured at single time-point, while our study considered time-dependent variations in the PUFA content by inclusion of the data from 3 consecutive examinations across the 10-years. Herein observed adverse EPA associations might be attributed to the aging of participants, an epidemiological context associated with increase in BP. EPA is a precursor of prostaglandins with limited vasodilatory properties and its physiological function might be outweighed by the natural course of aging. Further on, associations reflecting absolute changes with incremental EPA increase were relatively small. Subjects in the highest EPA tertile presented with only +2.92 and +1.94 mmHg higher SBP and DBP over the 10-years, respectively, in a multivariable-adjusted model. Of importance, baseline mean SBP/DBP was already higher (137/89 mmHg) and is with expected increasing trend over time due to aging, altogether potentially contributing to the observed 1.46 higher odds of being hypertensive with incremental EPA increase.

Our results should be interpreted in context of a population free of acute or chronic illnesses and residing in rapidly urbanizing areas. We showed raising hypertension prevalence across the 10-years, significant in rural areas. In urban dwellers we observed a non-significant decrease in hypertension rate, partly due to 10-years decline in both SBP and DBP of approximately 7 mmHg. Notably, 19.3% rural and 17.5% urban dwellers used hypertension medication at baseline. The number dramatically increased across the 10-years resulting in 35.7% and 33.1% of the respective subjects on medication in 2015, partly because study participants diagnosed with baseline high BP were instructed to their local clinics. Compliance with therapeutic protocols might be more prominent among urbans with readily available healthcare, resulting in a stabilization of hypertension prevalence across the 10-years. In our study, long-chain PUFA were not associated with status of hypertension across the 10-years, except for EPA being adversely related. Increased medication use might have masked the associations, due to the interaction with lipid metabolism [31]. The large-scale Atherosclerosis Risk in Communities study previously showed protective associations between total PUFA cholesterol ester content and 6-years prevalent and incident hypertension, with individual EPA and AA exhibiting adverse associations [32]. Overall, our results remain inconclusive on the association between fatty acids and hypertension status in the black South Africans, and larger cohorts should confirm the relationship.

The metabolic context of our results is of consideration. Within the sample of black South Africans, we found unusually high levels of long-chain PUFA in plasma phospholipids. Previously reported levels of serum AA were higher in African Americans with diabetes or metabolic syndrome, in comparison with their counterparts of European ancestry [33]. Still the levels were substantially lower (9.8 ± 1.9%) [33], in comparison with our study (mean range across the 10 years: 13.57–18.13%). In a larger population of Chinese subjects of similar age group as our participants, percentage of AA in total serum content was 6.02 ± 1.61 [12]. Also, in our study 10-years mean plasma phospholipid content of DHA exceeded 3.5%, which is above 2.5–3.4% previously reported in healthy populations [12,34–36]. Higher levels of long-chain AA and DHA observed herein might result from marked desaturase-6 activity. Observed DHA content is of special importance as only up to 1% of dietary ALA is endogenously converted to DHA [37] and our population had substantially low n-3 intake at baseline (year of 2005) [5] (median of 33 to 61 mg EPA +52 to 109 mg DHA below recommendations by FAO [38]). According to 2004 International Society for the Study of Fatty Acids and Lipids expert opinion, recommended combined EPA + DHA intake in general population should be at least 500 mg daily, conferring substantially low intake of the fatty acids in our subjects. A low fat, high carbohydrate diet is reported in other urbanizing populations [39] and is associated with augmented fatty acid synthesis [40]. We thus speculate that restricted intake of n-3 rich food in the black South Africans might be a conditional metabolic factor enhancing desaturase activity towards physiologically active long-chain plasma products, including AA and DHA. Notably, in our study baseline intake of marine PUFA was not correlated with its plasma phospholipid status. Previous results in 1834 Chinese community dwellers demonstrated strong correlation among erythrocyte long-chain n-3 content and their dietary counterparts [30]. However, when we evaluated n-3 intake as sum of preformed EPA, DHA and plant-originated ALA we observed a direct correlation with status of EPA (r = 0.138, p = 0.017) and DHA (r = 0.218, p = 0.000). The latter suggests that in our subjects, dietary ALA is pronouncedly converted towards plasma long-chain products by activity of desaturase enzymes. Previous reports indicate specific FADS genetic make-up in populations of African descent. Results from the Diabetes Heart Study showed that 81% of African Americans are carriers of FADS rs174537 variant [33], associated with AA, eicosadienoic acid and EPA levels [41]. We suggest that historically low intake of n-3 PUFA in the population of black South Africans is coupled with genetically-regulated higher metabolic conversion towards AA and DHA.

We showed inverse associations of AA with BP across the 10-years. Observational studies found plasma AA to be protectively associated with coronary heart disease [42,43] and type 2 diabetes risk [44]. AA is a precursor of eicosanoids with pro-inflammatory properties and vasomodulatory function [45]. AA is also a precursor of epoxydes with anti-vasodilatory function, mediated by soluble epoxyde hydrolase [46]. A favourable balance between n-3 and n-6 intake potentiates production of vasodilatory eiocosanoids from AA and decreases BP [45,46]. Herein observed protective relationship of AA might be due to metabolic adaptation conditional to a historically low n-3 long-chain PUFA intake. The associations of AA were prominent within urban dwellers, potentially due to the interaction with micronutrient intake, such as magnesium known to influence desaturase-6 function [47]. In a previous cross-sectional study of 2447 middle-aged and older Chinese community dwellers, AA exhibited neutral associations with BP, but study subjects in the highest tertile of serum DHA had significantly lower SBP and DBP in comparison with those in the lowest [12]. Although there was an inverse trend, DHA was not significantly associated with BP, potentially due to limited size of our study sample. It is possible that in our population with inherently low n-3 PUFA intake, extensive conversion to DHA underpins its incorporation in phospholipid cellular bilayers for non-vascular beneficial effects. Prospective analysis among 381 healthy, middle-aged and elderly subjects participating in the Kuopio Ischemic Heart Disease Risk Factor study also failed to demonstrate associations between individual long-chain n-3 serum PUFA and BP over 10 years [48].

We observed protective associations of osbond acid with BP. Dietary contribution to osbond acid status is negligible and its physiological role is due to metabolic conversion. To our knowledge, no previous study reported associations of osbond acid with clinical outcomes. In our study, the 10-year increase in n-6 AA and osbond acid were related to clinically relevant 3–4 mmHg lower BP for subjects within the highest tertile of the PUFA content. The protective associations might reflect pronounced utilization of the n-6 long-chain products for physiological function in this population with restricted n-3 intake. The suggestion to increase n-6 intake however remains a controversial approach [49–51] and previous studies suggest neutral effects from increased n-6 intake to BP lowering [52,53]. As intake of essential n-6 linoleic acid (C18:3 n-6) and n-3 ALA are highly correlated since both are abundant in plant oils, observed inverse associations might reflect beneficial implications of higher intake of dietary ALA itself and its metabolic products [46,54].

Finally, our results should be placed in the context of a population under urbanisation coupled with transitions in nutritional habits. The protective 10-year associations of AA and osbond acid remained significant in urban dwellers only. In urban subjects only we observed decrease in EPA and DHA in plasma phospholipids, possibly be due to westernised dietary patterns characterized by cooking oils rich in linoleic acid and n-6 PUFA [55] and poor intake of n-3 sources (such as whole grains, vegetables and marine food). The finding on EPA and DHA decrease thus supports existing policies on increasing *n*-3 intake in this population undergoing urbanisation [56]. In rural subjects only we observed an increase in DHA, which was also associated with lower DBP. It is less plausible that the increase was due to pronounced intake of DHA from marine food, rather a consequence of enhanced conversion towards long-chain *n*-3 products within rural subjects with significantly lower *n*-3 intake.

Lack of consistent association between plasma *n*-3 PUFA and BP in our study is partly in line with recent findings from ASCEND trial conducted in 16,000 diabetic middle-aged and older subjects [57]. The authors demonstrated no beneficial effects of daily consumption of *n*-3 fish oil capsules (460 mg EPA + 380 mg DHA) in comparison with placebo olive oil, and regarding incidence of serious vascular events upon 7.4 years follow-up [57]. On the other hand, REDUCE-IT showed that among 8000 patients with elevated triglycerides and stable LDL-cholesterol, receiving 2 g of highly purified EPA ethyl ester twice daily was associated with significantly lower risk of composite cardiovascular event, in comparison with placebo and despite the use of statins [58]. Based upon our results and considering the low *n*-3 PUFA intake [5] we may not discard the role of dietary *n*-3 PUFA and particularly EPA in strategies towards BP optimisation in Africa, and future intervention studies with increasing *n*-3 intake should elucidate the relationship.

The strength of our study lays in a repeated-measures design, evaluating time-dependent changes in BP and hypertension related to fat intake and metabolism. Furthermore, urbanisation-specific analyses and inclusion of a panel of demographic and clinical confounders provide robustness to the obtained relationships. We reported dietary and fat intake profiles across urbanisation categories in line with previously reported baseline dietary intake for the complete cohort (n 1950) [5] implying generalizability of our results to the population of black South Africans. Herein reported plasma fatty acid profiles are comparable to recent report within larger sample (n 711) [18] of the same cohort of black South Africans participating PURE, outweighing potential concern on the limited sample size of 300 subjects. Of note, 10-year attrition rate might have blurred some of the associations. However, we applied longitudinal analysis accounting for time-dependent variation of outcomes and exposures, providing additional reliability to the observed associations. We followed no changes in usage of medication or any other lifestyle confounder, potentially limiting our results. Although we accounted for an array of structured lifestyle, demographic and clinical confounders, the residual confounding cannot be ruled out.

In conclusion, our data advocate for a link between fat intake, blood pressure and urbanisation in a population of black South Africans with historically low omega-3 intake. Ten-year hypertension prevalence increased in the 300 subjects and only in urban residents did we observe a tendency towards 10-year optimization of hypertension status. Regardless of urbanisation areas there was an increase in individual plasma *n*-6 PUFA over 10 years, but only in urbans there was a decrease in EPA and DHA status, supporting policies on *n*-3 dietary reinforcement. The individual *n*-6 PUFA were inversely associated with blood pressure, prominently within urban dwellers. Taken together the results imply a protective mechanism linked with fat metabolism and vascular health in black South African population undergoing rapid nutritional transition. Indicated population-specific metabotype in black South Africans is possibly linked with genetic background and further research on FADS1 and FADS2 variants, desaturase activity and association with vascular function is warranted in the population.

Supplementary Materials: The following are available online at http://www.mdpi.com/2304-8158/8/9/394/s1, Figure S1: Flow-diagram explaining selection of the 300 black South Africans for the longitudinal analysis of associations between fatty acids and blood pressure over 10 years, Table S1: Blood pressure across 10 years in black South Africans, Table S2: Plasma phospholipids fatty acid status across 10-years in rural (n 140) and urban (n 160) black South Africans, Table S3: Baseline correlations between dietary intake of *n*-3 fatty acids and long-chain fatty acids in plasma phospholipids in 300 black South Africans: Pearson correlation matrix, Table S4: Ten-year associations between plasma phospholipid long-chain fatty acids and blood pressure in rural and urban black South Africans, Table S5: Ten-year associations between plasma phospholipid long-chain fatty acids and hypertension status in black South Africans.

Author Contributions: Conceptualization, M.M.Z., A.E.S. and C.M.S.; Methodology, M.M.Z., A.E.S., C.R., J.B. and C.M.S.; Software, M.M.Z. and C.R.; Formal analysis, M.M.Z.; Investigation, M.M.Z., A.E.S., J.B., I.M.K. and

C.M.S.; Resources, A.E.S. and C.M.S.; Data curation, M.M.Z. and C.R.; Writing—original draft preparation, M.M.Z.; Writing—review and editing, M.M.Z., A.E.S., J.B. and C.M.S.; Visualization, M.M.Z.; Supervision, A.E.S. and C.M.S.; Project administration, I.M.K., A.E.S. and C.M.S.; Funding acquisition, A.E.S. and C.M.S.

Funding: This research was funded by SANPAD (South Africa Netherlands Research Programme on Alternatives in Development), South African National Research Foundation [NRF GUN numbers 2069139 and FA2006040700010], North-West University, Potchefstroom, South Africa, SASA [South African Sugar Association, Project 228], Roche Diagnostics South Africa, and the Population Health Research Institute, ON, Canada and the South African Medical Research Council. Any opinion, findings, and conclusions or recommendations expressed in this material are those of the authors, and therefore, the NRF does not accept any liability in this regard.

Acknowledgments: We would like to acknowledge the PURE South Africa team: A Kruger, PURE-SA research team, field workers and office staff in the Africa Unit for Transdisciplinary Health Research (AUTHeR), Faculty of Health Sciences, North-West University, Potchefstroom, South Africa. The PURE International: S Yusuf and the PURE project office staff at the Population Health Research Institute, Hamilton Health Sciences and McMaster University. ON, Canada.

Conflicts of Interest: The authors declare no conflict of interest.

References

1. Popkin, B.M. Nutrition in transition: The changing global nutrition challenge. *Asia Pac. J. Clin. Nutr.* **2001**, *10*, S13–S18. [CrossRef]
2. Alsheikh-Ali, A.A.; Omar, M.I.; Raal, F.J.; Rashed, W.; Hamoui, O.; Kane, A.; Alami, M.; Abreu, P.; Mashhoud, W.M. Cardiovascular risk factor burden in Africa and the Middle East: The Africa Middle East Cardiovascular Epidemiological (ACE) study. *PLoS ONE* **2014**, *9*, e102830. [CrossRef]
3. Danaei, G.; Finucane, M.M.; Lin, J.K.; Singh, G.M.; Paciorek, C.J.; Cowan, M.J.; Farzadfar, F.; Stevens, G.A.; Lim, S.S.; Riley, L.M.; et al. Global Burden of Metabolic Risk Factors of Chronic Diseases Collaborating Group (Blood Pressure). National, regional, and global trends in systolic blood pressure since 1980: Systematic analysis of health examination surveys and epidemiological studies with 786 country-years and 5.4 million participants. *Lancet* **2011**, *377*, 568–577.
4. Schutte, A.E.; Schutte, R.; Huisman, H.W.; van Rooyen, J.M.; Fourie, C.M.; Malan, N.T.; Malan, L.; Mels, C.M.; Smith, W.; Moss, S.J.; et al. Are behavioural risk factors to be blamed for the conversion from optimal blood pressure to hypertensive status in Black South Africans? A 5-year prospective study. *Int. J. Epidemiol.* **2012**, *41*, 1114–1123. [CrossRef]
5. Richter, M.; Baumgartner, J.; Wentzel-Viljoen, E.; Smuts, C.M. Different dietary fatty acids are associated with blood lipids in healthy South African men and women: The PURE study. *Int. J. Cardiol.* **2014**, *172*, 368–374. [CrossRef]
6. Bagge, C.N.; Strandhave, C.; Skov, C.M.; Svensson, M.; Schmidt, E.B.; Christensen, J.H. Marine n-3 polyunsaturated fatty acids affect the blood pressure control in patients with newly diagnosed hypertension–a 1-year follow-up study. *Nutr. Res.* **2017**, *38*, 71–78. [CrossRef]
7. Mozaffarian, D.; Wu, J.H. Omega-3 fatty acids and cardiovascular disease: Effects on risk factors, molecular pathways, and clinical events. *J. Am. Coll. Cardiol.* **2011**, *58*, 2047–2067. [CrossRef]
8. Archer, E.; Blair, S.N. Implausible data, false memories, and the status quo in dietary assessment. *Adv. Nutr.* **2015**, *6*, 229–230. [CrossRef]
9. Ma, J.; Folsom, A.R.; Shahar, E.; Eckfeldt, J.H. Plasma fatty acid composition as an indicator of habitual dietary fat intake in middle-aged adults. The Atherosclerosis Risk in Communities (ARIC) Study Investigators. *Am. J. Clin. Nutr.* **1995**, *62*, 564–571. [CrossRef]
10. Jackson, K.H.; Harris, W.S. Blood Fatty Acid Profiles: New Biomarkers for Cardiometabolic Disease Risk. *Curr. Atheroscler. Rep.* **2018**, *20*, 22. [CrossRef]
11. Liu, Q.; Matthan, N.R.; Manson, J.E.; Howard, B.V.; Tinker, L.F.; Neuhouser, M.L.; Van Horn, L.V.; Rossouw, J.E.; Allison, M.A.; Martin, L.W.; et al. Plasma Phospholipid Fatty Acids and Coronary Heart Disease Risk: A Matched Case-Control Study within the Women's Health Initiative Observational Study. *Nutrients* **2019**, *11*, 1672. [CrossRef]
12. Yang, B.; Ding, F.; Yan, J.; Ye, X.W.; Xu, X.L.; Wang, F.L.; Yu, W. Exploratory serum fatty acid patterns associated with blood pressure in community-dwelling middle-aged and elderly Chinese. *Lipids Health Dis.* **2016**, *15*, 58. [CrossRef]

13. Simon, J.A.; Fong, J.; Bernert, J.T., Jr. Serum fatty acids and blood pressure. *Hypertension* **1996**, *27*, 303–307. [CrossRef]
14. Grimsgaard, S.; Bonaa, K.H.; Jacobsen, B.K.; Bjerve, K.S. Plasma saturated and linoleic fatty acids are independently associated with blood pressure. *Hypertension* **1999**, *34*, 478–483. [CrossRef]
15. Virtanen, J.K.; Nyantika, A.N.; Kauhanen, J.; Voutilainen, S.; Tuomainen, T.P. Serum long-chain n-3 polyunsaturated fatty acids, methylmercury and blood pressure in an older population. *Hypertens. Res.* **2012**, *35*, 1000–1004. [CrossRef]
16. Liu, J.C.; Conklin, S.M.; Manuck, S.B.; Yao, J.K.; Muldoon, M.F. Long-chain omega-3 fatty acids and blood pressure. *Am. J. Hypertens.* **2011**, *24*, 1121–1126. [CrossRef]
17. Yang, B.; Ding, F.; Wang, F.L.; Yan, J.; Ye, X.W.; Yu, W.; Li, D. Association of serum fatty acid and estimated desaturase activity with hypertension in middle-aged and elderly Chinese population. *Sci. Rep.* **2016**, *6*, 23446. [CrossRef]
18. Ojwang, A.A.; Kruger, H.S.; Zec, M.; Ricci, C.; Pieters, M.; Kruger, I.M.; Wentzel-Viljoen, E.; Smuts, C.M. Plasma phospholipid fatty acid patterns are associated with adiposity and the metabolic syndrome in black South Africans: A cross-sectional study. *Cardiovasc. J. Afr.* **2019**, *30*, 1–11.
19. Teo, K.; Chow, C.K.; Vaz, M.; Rangarajan, S.; Yusuf, S. PURE Investigators-Writing Group. The Prospective Urban Rural Epidemiology (PURE) study: Examining the impact of societal influences on chronic noncommunicable diseases in low-, middle-, and high-income countries. *Am. Heart J.* **2009**, *158*, 1–7. [CrossRef]
20. Baumgartner, J.; Smuts, C.M.; Malan, L.; Kvalsvig, J.; van Stuijvenberg, M.E.; Hurrell, R.F.; Zimmermann, M.B. Effects of iron and n-3 fatty acid supplementation, alone and in combination, on cognition in school children: A randomized, double-blind, placebo-controlled intervention in South Africa. *Am. J. Clin. Nutr.* **2012**, *96*, 1327–1338. [CrossRef]
21. Folch, J.; Lees, M.; Sloane Stanley, G.H. A simple method for the isolation and purification of total lipides from animal tissues. *J. Biol. Chem.* **1957**, *226*, 497–509.
22. Williams, B.; Mancia, G.; Spiering, W.; Agabiti Rosei, E.; Azizi, M.; Burnier, M.; Clement, D.L.; Coca, A.; de Simone, G.; Dominiczak, A.; et al. 2018 ESC/ESH Guidelines for the management of arterial hypertension: The Task Force for the management of arterial hypertension of the European Society of Cardiology and the European Society of Hypertension: The Task Force for the management of arterial hypertension of the European Society of Cardiology and the European Society of Hypertension. *J. Hypertens.* **2018**, *36*, 1953–2041.
23. Kruger, H.S.; Venter, C.S.; Vorster, H.H.; Margetts, B.M. Physical inactivity is the major determinant of obesity in black women in the North West Province, South Africa: The THUSA study. Transition and Health During Urbanisation of South Africa. *Nutrition* **2002**, *18*, 422–427. [CrossRef]
24. Wentzel-Viljoen, E.; Laubscher, R.; Kruger, A. Using different approaches to assess the reproducibility of a culturally sensitive quantified food frequency questionnaire. *S. Afr. J. Clin. Nutr.* **2011**, *24*, 143–148. [CrossRef]
25. Davis, C.; Bryan, J.; Hodgson, J.; Murphy, K. Definition of the Mediterranean diet; a literature review. *Nutrients* **2015**, *7*, 9139–9153. [CrossRef]
26. Tucker, L.A. Fiber Intake and Insulin Resistance in 6374 Adults: The Role of Abdominal Obesity. *Nutrients* **2018**, *10*, 237. [CrossRef]
27. Toyama, K.; Nishioka, T.; Isshiki, A.; Ando, T.; Inoue, Y.; Kirimura, M.; Kamiyama, T.; Sasaki, O.; Ito, H.; Maruyama, Y.; et al. Eicosapentaenoic acid combined with optimal statin therapy improves endothelial dysfunction in patients with coronary artery disease. *Cardiovasc. Drugs Ther.* **2014**, *28*, 53–59. [CrossRef]
28. Sasaki, J.; Miwa, T.; Odawara, M. Administration of highly purified eicosapentaenoic acid to statin-treated diabetic patients further improves vascular function. *Endocr. J.* **2012**, *59*, 297–304. [CrossRef]
29. Bäck, M.; Hansson, G.K. Omega-3 fatty acids, cardiovascular risk, and the resolution of inflammation. *FASEB J.* **2019**, *33*, 1536–1539. [CrossRef]
30. Zeng, F.F.; Sun, L.L.; Liu, Y.H.; Xu, Y.; Guan, K.; Ling, W.H.; Chen, Y.M. Higher Erythrocyte n–3 PUFAs Are Associated with Decreased Blood Pressure in Middle-Aged and Elderly Chinese Adults–3. *J. Nutr.* **2014**, *144*, 1240–1246. [CrossRef]
31. Puzyrenko, A.M.; Chekman, I.S.; Briuzhina, T.S.; Horchakova, N.O. Influence of antihypertensive and metabolic drugs on fatty acids content of lipids in cardiomyocytes of rats with spontaneous hypertension. *Ukr. Kyi Biokhimichnyi Zhurnal (1999)* **2013**, *85*, 67–74. [CrossRef]

32. Zheng, Z.J.; Folsom, A.R.; Ma, J.; Arnett, D.K.; McGovern, P.G.; Eckfeldt, J.H. ARIC Study Investigators. Plasma fatty acid composition and 6-year incidence of hypertension in middle-aged adults: The Atherosclerosis Risk in Communities (ARIC) Study. *Am. J. Epidemiol.* **1999**, *150*, 492–500. [CrossRef]
33. Sergeant, S.; Hugenschmidt, C.E.; Rudock, M.E.; Ziegler, J.T.; Ivester, P.; Ainsworth, H.C.; Vaidya, D.; Case, L.D.; Langefeld, C.D.; Freedman, B.I.; et al. Differences in arachidonic acid levels and fatty acid desaturase (FADS) gene variants in African Americans and European Americans with diabetes or the metabolic syndrome. *Br. J. Nutr.* **2012**, *107*, 547–555. [CrossRef]
34. Conquer, J.A.; Martin, J.B.; Tummon, I.; Watson, L.; Tekpetey, F. Fatty acid analysis of blood serum, seminal plasma, and spermatozoa of normozoospermic vs. asthenozoospermic Men. *Lipids* **1999**, *34*, 793–799. [CrossRef]
35. Laidlaw, M.; Holub, B.J. Effects of supplementation with fish oil-derived n-3 fatty acids and gamma-linolenic acid on circulating plasma lipids and fatty acid profiles in women. *Am. J. Clin. Nutr.* **2003**, *77*, 37–42. [CrossRef]
36. Young, G.S.; Maharaj, N.J.; Conquer, J.A. Blood phospholipid fatty acid analysis of adults with and without attention deficit/hyperactivity disorder. *Lipids* **2004**, *39*, 117–123. [CrossRef]
37. Brenna, J.T.; Salem, N., Jr.; Sinclair, A., Jr.; Cunnane, S.C. Alpha-linolenic acid supplementation and conversion to n-3 long-chain polyunsaturated fatty acids in humans. *Prostaglandins Leukot. Essent. Fat. Acids* **2009**, *80*, 85–91. [CrossRef]
38. Elmadfa, I.; Kornsteiner, M. Fats and fatty acid requirements for adults. *Ann. Nutr. Metab.* **2009**, *55*, 56. [CrossRef]
39. Vessby, B.; Ahrén, B.; Warensjö, E.; Lindgärde, F. Plasma lipid fatty acid composition, desaturase activities and insulin sensitivity in Amerindian women. *Nutr. Metab. Cardiovasc. Dis.* **2012**, *22*, 176–181. [CrossRef]
40. King, I.B.; Lemaitre, R.N.; Kestin, M. Effect of a low-fat diet on fatty acid composition in red cells, plasma phospholipids, and cholesterol esters: Investigation of a biomarker of total fat intake. *Am. J. Clin. Nutr.* **2006**, *83*, 227–236. [CrossRef]
41. Tanaka, T.; Shen, J.; Abecasis, G.R.; Kisialiou, A.; Ordovas, J.M.; Guralnik, J.M.; Singleton, A.; Bandinelli, S.; Cherubini, A.; Arnett, D.; et al. Genome-wide association study of plasma polyunsaturated fatty acids in the InCHIANTI Study. *PLoS Genet.* **2009**, *5*, e1000338. [CrossRef]
42. Wang, L.; Folsom, A.R.; Eckfeldt, J.H. Plasma fatty acid composition and incidence of coronary heart disease in middle aged adults: The Atherosclerosis Risk in Communities (ARIC) Study. *Nutr. Metab. Cardiovasc. Dis.* **2003**, *13*, 256–266. [CrossRef]
43. Salonen, J.T.; Salonen, R.; Penttila, I.; Herranen, J.; Jauhiainen, M.; Kantola, M.; Lappetelainen, R.; Maenpaa, P.H.; Alfthan, G.; Puska, P. Serum fatty acids, apolipoproteins, selenium and vitamin antioxidants and the risk of death from coronary artery disease. *Am. J. Cardiol.* **1985**, *56*, 226–231. [CrossRef]
44. Yary, T.; Voutilainen, S.; Tuomainen, T.P.; Ruusunen, A.; Nurmi, T.; Virtanen, J.K. Serum n-6 polyunsaturated fatty acids, delta5- and delta6-destaurase activities, and risk of incident type 2 diabetes in men: The Kuopio Ischaemic Heart Disease Risk Factor Study. *Am. J. Clin. Nutr.* **2016**, *103*, 1337–1343. [CrossRef]
45. Sonnweber, T.; Pizzini, A.; Nairz, M.; Weiss, G.; Tancevski, I. Arachidonic Acid Metabolites in Cardiovascular and Metabolic Diseases. *Int. J. Mol. Sci.* **2018**, *19*, 3285. [CrossRef]
46. Caligiuri, S.P.; Aukema, H.M.; Ravandi, A.; Guzman, R.; Dibrov, E.; Pierce, G.N. Flaxseed consumption reduces blood pressure in patients with hypertension by altering circulating oxylipins via an α-linolenic acid–induced inhibition of soluble epoxide hydrolase. *Hypertension* **2014**, *64*, 53–59. [CrossRef]
47. Das, U.N. Nutritional factors in the pathobiology of human essential hypertension. *Nutrition* **2001**, *17*, 337–346. [CrossRef]
48. Nyantika, A.N.; Tuomainen, T.P.; Kauhanen, J.; Voutilainen, S.; Virtanen, J.K. Serum long-chain omega-3 polyunsaturated fatty acids and future blood pressure in an ageing population. *J. Nutr. Health Aging* **2015**, *19*, 498–503. [CrossRef]
49. US Department of Health and Human Services and US Department of Agriculture. 2015–2020 Dietary Guidelines for Americans (DGA), 8th. ed. December 2015. Available online: http://health.gov/dietaryguidelines/2015/guidelines/ (accessed on 29 March 2019).

50. Sacks, F.M.; Lichtenstein, A.H.; Wu, J.H.Y.; Appel, L.J.; Creager, M.A.; Kris-Etherton, P.M.; Miller, M.; Rimm, E.B.; Rudel, L.L.; Robinson, J.G.; et al. American Heart Association. Dietary fats and cardiovascular disease: A Presidential Advisory from the American Heart Association. *Circulation* **2017**, *136*, e1–e23. [CrossRef]
51. Nettleton, J.A.; von Schacky, C.; Brouwer, I.A.; Koletzko, B. International Society for the Study of Fatty Acids and Lipids 2016 debate: For science based dietary guidelines on fats, meta-analysis and systematic reviews are decisive. *Ann. Nutr. Metab.* **2017**, *71*, 26–30. [CrossRef]
52. Al-Khudairy, L.; Hartley, L.; Clar, C.; Flowers, N.; Hooper, L.; Rees, K. Omega-6 fatty acids for the primary prevention of cardiovascular disease. *Cochrane Database Syst. Rev.* **2015**, *16*, CD011094. [CrossRef]
53. Vafeiadou, K.; Weech, M.; Altowaijri, H.; Todd, S.; Yaqoob, P.; Jackson, K.G.; Lovegrove, J.A. Replacement of saturated with unsaturated fats had no impact on vascular function but beneficial effects on lipid biomarkers, E-selectin, and blood pressure: Results from the randomized, controlled Dietary Intervention and VAScular function (DIVAS) study. *Am. J. Clin. Nutr.* **2015**, *102*, 40–48. [CrossRef]
54. Maki, K.C.; Eren, F.; Cassens, M.E.; Dicklin, M.R.; Davidson, M.H. ω-6 Polyunsaturated Fatty Acids and Cardiometabolic Health: Current Evidence, Controversies, and Research Gaps. *Adv. Nutr.* **2018**, *9*, 688–700. [CrossRef]
55. Chilton, F.H.; Murphy, R.C.; Wilson, B.A.; Sergeant, S.; Ainsworth, H.; Seeds, M.C.; Mathias, R.A. Diet-gene interactions and PUFA metabolism: A potential contributor to health disparities and human diseases. *Nutrients* **2014**, *6*, 1993–2022. [CrossRef]
56. Smuts, C.M.; Wolmarans, P. The importance of the quality or type of fat in the diet: A food-based dietary guideline for South Africa. *S. Afr. J. Clin. Nutr.* **2013**, *26*, S87–S99.
57. ASCEND Study Collaborative, Group; Bowman, L.; Mafham, M.; Wallendszus, K.; Stevens, W.; Buck, G.; Barton, J.; Murphy, K.; Aung, T.; Haynes, R.; et al. Effects of n-3 fatty acid supplements in diabetes mellitus. *N. Engl. J. Med.* **2018**, *379*, 1540–1550. [CrossRef]
58. Bhatt, D.L.; Steg, P.G.; Miller, M.; Brinton, E.A.; Jacobson, T.A.; Ketchum, S.B.; Doyle, R.T., Jr.; Juliano, R.A.; Jiao, L.; Granowitz, C.; et al. Cardiovascular risk reduction with icosapent ethyl for hypertriglyceridemia. *N. Engl. J. Med.* **2019**, *380*, 11–22. [CrossRef]

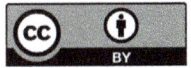

© 2019 by the authors. Licensee MDPI, Basel, Switzerland. This article is an open access article distributed under the terms and conditions of the Creative Commons Attribution (CC BY) license (http://creativecommons.org/licenses/by/4.0/).

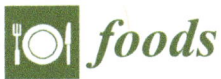

Review

Bioactive Candy: Effects of Licorice on the Cardiovascular System

Mikkel R. Deutch [1], Daniela Grimm [1,2,3], Markus Wehland [2], Manfred Infanger [2] and Marcus Krüger [2,*]

1. Department of Biomedicine, Aarhus University, 8000 Aarhus C, Denmark; mikkelrd@gmail.com (M.R.D.); dgg@biomed.au.dk (D.G.)
2. Clinic for Plastic, Aesthetic and Hand Surgery, Otto von Guericke University, 39120 Magdeburg, Germany; markus.wehland@med.ovgu.de (M.W.); manfred.infanger@med.ovgu.de (M.I.)
3. Gravitational Biology and Translational Regenerative Medicine, Faculty of Medicine and Mechanical Engineering, Otto von Guericke University, 39120 Magdeburg, Germany
* Correspondence: marcus.krueger@med.ovgu.de; Tel.: +49-391-67-21267

Received: 24 September 2019; Accepted: 9 October 2019; Published: 14 October 2019

Abstract: Licorice, today chiefly utilized as a flavoring additive in tea, tobacco and candy, is one of the oldest used herbs for medicinal purposes and consists of up to 300 active compounds. The main active constituent of licorice is the prodrug glycyrrhizin, which is successively converted to 3β-monoglucuronyl-18β-glycyrrhetinic acid (3MGA) and 18β-glycyrrhetinic acid (GA) in the intestines. Despite many reported health benefits, 3MGA and GA inhibit the 11-β-hydrogenase type II enzyme (11β-HSD2) oxidizing cortisol to cortisone. Through activation of mineralocorticoid receptors, high cortisol levels induce a mild form of apparent mineralocorticoid excess in the kidney and increase systemic vascular resistance. Continuous inhibition of 11β-HSD2 related to excess licorice consumption will create a state of hypernatremia, hypokalemia and increased fluid volume, which can cause serious life-threatening complications especially in patients already suffering from cardiovascular diseases. Two recent meta-analyses of 18 and 26 studies investigating the correlation between licorice intake and blood pressure revealed statistically significant increases both in systolic (5.45 mmHg) and in diastolic blood pressure (3.19/1.74 mmHg). This review summarizes and evaluates current literature about the acute and chronic effects of licorice ingestion on the cardiovascular system with special focus on blood pressure. Starting from the molecular actions of licorice (metabolites) inside the cells, it describes how licorice intake is affecting the human body and shows the boundaries between the health benefits of licorice and possible harmful effects.

Keywords: licorice; glycyrrhizin; glycyrrhetinic acid; glabridin; 11-β-dehydrogenase isozyme 2; hyperaldosteronism; hypokalemia; hypertension

---

1. The Sweet "Father of Herbal Medicine"

Licorice is the root of the legume *Glycyrrhiza glabra* (Figure 1a) that grows in varieties in warm areas like the Middle East, Asia and Southern Europe. It is one of the oldest used herbs in ancient medicine and referred to as "the father of herbal medicine" [1]. Licorice, from which a sweet flavor can be extracted, has been used in herbal and traditional medicine in both Eastern and Western cultures dating back to beyond 4000 BC [2]. The early Egyptians and Assyrians are known to have cultivated the 'sweet root' that was later imported to China, where it has been used for centuries under the name '*Gan Cao*' [3]. It has also been described by ancient Greeks, including Hippocrates and Theophrastus, as well as by Romans [2,4]. Today, the Scandinavian countries seem to have the most consumers of licorice; however, licorice intake is also a popular strategy to quench thirst during Ramadan (based on its historical utilization in the desert or on battlefields, where travelers and soldiers drank licorice extracts to combat thirst sensation on long marches). Although the main active compound glycyrrhizin is considered to be 50-times sweeter than sucrose [5], licorice is rarely used for sweetening purposes alone due to its associated flavor and the brownish color that would be imparted to non-acidic foods [2,6]. Since the 18th century, the primary use comprises mainly licorice extracts (in pharmacy called *Succus liquiritae*) as a flavoring additive in tea, tobacco, candy (Figure 1b) and other sweets, but the licorice root itself (*Liquiritae radix*) is still used as a dietary supplement in some parts of the world [7]. Among people preferring alternative or complementary medicine, historical uses for licorice were revived and are still practiced today [8–10].

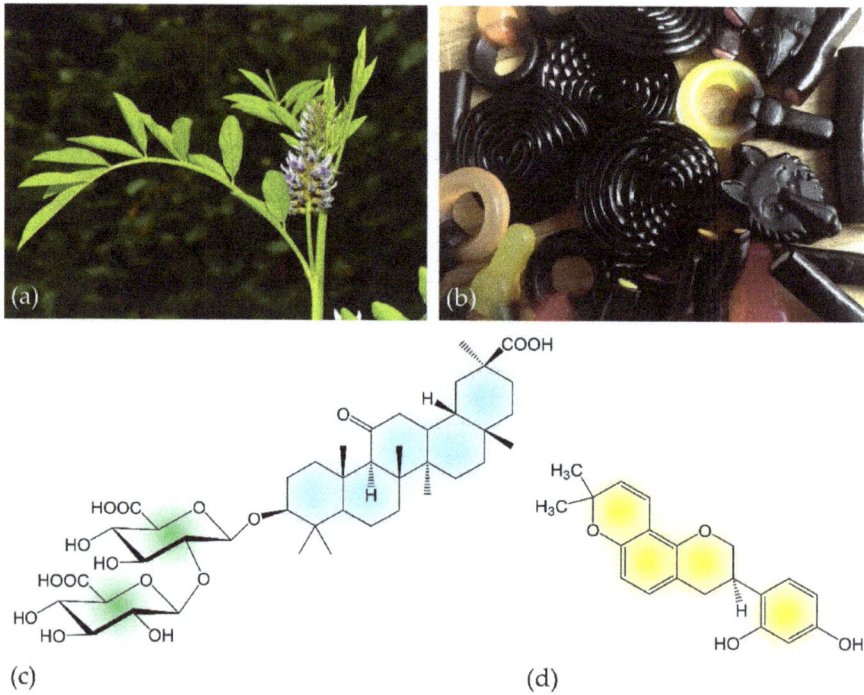

Figure 1. (a) Inflorescence of *Glycyrrhiza glabra* L.; (b) licorice-containing candies; (c) chemical structure of the prodrug glycyrrhizin ($C_{42}H_{62}O_{16}$), the main active compound of licorice. The molecule consists of two molecules of glucuronic acid (left) that are linked to 18β-glycyrrhetinic acid; (d) chemical structure of glabridin ($C_{20}H_{20}O_4$), a further bioactive licorice compound. Colors indicate molecule structures used in following schematics.

On the one hand, the health benefits ascribed to licorice are numerous: for centuries it has been used in herbal and folk medicine to treat multiple diseases such as gastrointestinal symptoms and respiratory diseases [10]. The broad spectrum of activities known today comprises immunostimulatory and anti-ulcer effects [11–13], anti-viral and anti-microbial effects [14,15], hepatoprotective [16,17], anti-carcinogenic [18] and several other positive effects that contribute to the protection of the nervous, respiratory, endocrine and cardiovascular system [9]. Licorice is also effective against gastrointestinal problems by repairing the inner layer of the stomach and cleansing the respiratory system by increasing the production of mucus. Furthermore, other extracts of the licorice root have been tested in the treatment of gastritis induced by *Helicobacter pylori* and showed promising results [19,20]. The polyphenolic flavonoid glabridin possesses hypoglycemic effects by modulating glucose and lipid metabolism [21,22], similar to effects attributed to green tea extract [23]. On the other hand, it is well-known that consuming excessive quantities of licorice can impact upon cardiometabolic health by elevating blood pressure (BP), and thus, may be a cause of hypertension and other cardiovascular complications [24–30].

Hypertension is one of the major concerns for our healthcare system and was the leading contributor to premature death in 2015 [31]. Due to the higher arterial BP, it has been proven to be a major risk factor of cardiovascular diseases (CVD). The global prevalence of hypertension was estimated to be about 1.13 billion. Generally, hypertension is the cut-off BP value, where the benefits of treatment outweigh the associated risks. According to the European Society of Cardiology (ESC) "hypertension" is defined as a systolic BP ≥ 140 mmHg and a diastolic BP ≥ 90 mmHg [32]. Hypertension is divided into primary and secondary forms. It is a multifactorial disease, where the contribution of different factors is variable and with a small effect size. Most of the patients have no clear etiology, and they are classified as having primary hypertension. According to Charles et al. [33], about 5–10% of hypertensive patients have secondary hypertension, a result of a different disease affecting the cardiovascular system, such as renal diseases, primary hyperaldosteronism or obstructive sleep apnea.

Licorice and other drugs affecting the hormonal regulation of the water and electrolyte balance could be causing primary hypertension. To examine the actual cause of hypertension, some tests are needed. This would include measurements of plasma aldosterone and plasma renin. Aside from licorice, plenty of additional risk factors increase the possibility of developing hypertension [32].

In this review, we summarized and evaluated current literature about the effects of licorice ingestion on the cardiovascular system with special focus on BP. The literature was primarily identified using online databases. The search was completed on 24/9/2019. The primary registers included PubMed, Embase and ClinicalTrials.gov. Keywords that were used in the search included both "licorice" and "liquorice". Both variations were used to ensure a more complete search, since "licorice" is widely used in American literature whereas "liquorice" is common in British literature. In PubMed, the search for "liquorice" alone gave 4347 results, while "liquorice and hypertension" narrowed it down to 364 results. "Liquorice and cardiovascular disease" gave 379 results; "*Glycyrrhiza* and hypertension" resulted in 255 hits. We thoroughly collected information about the molecular and physiological mechanisms of licorice in order to explore the effects and prevalence of licorice intake in general. This way, we want to show the boundaries between its health benefits and possible harmful effects.

2. Pharmacological Effects of Licorice

2.1. Licorice Digestion and Chemistry of Metabolites

Licorice consists of up to 300 active compounds comprising phenolic acids, flavonoids, flavans, chalcones, isoflavans (including glabridin, the main compound found in the hydrophobic fraction of licorice extract) and isoflavonoids [10]. A species-dependent content of 3 to 5% the triterpenoid saponin glycyrrhizin (Figure 1c) accounts for the sweet taste of licorice root and is the main active constituent of licorice [6,34]. Although the presence of glycyrrhizin in licorice has been known for over 200 years, detailed chemical investigations have not been conducted until the mid of the 20th century [35]. In the licorice root, tribasic glycyrrhizin naturally occurs in form of its calcium and potassium salts. After oral ingestion, glycyrrhizin (which itself possesses only poor oral bioavailability) is successively hydrolyzed to 3β-monoglucuronyl-18β-glycyrrhetinic acid (3MGA) and the aglycone 18β-glycyrrhetinic acid (GA; also known as enoxolone) by intestinal bacteria possessing specialized β-glucuronidases [36,37]. GA is often considered as the active metabolite of licorice [38–40], but its pharmacokinetics seem to be more complex. After rapid absorption from the gut, 3MGA and GA circulate in the bloodstream. From there, they are transported to the liver by carrier molecules, where they are metabolized (Figure 2). In humans, hepatic processing is not yet clearly defined, but it is apparent that each metabolite can undergo further conjugation or reduction followed by biliary excretion [6]. The products are likely re-metabolized by the gut microbiome and thereby subjected to enterohepatic recycling requiring several days for complete elimination [41].

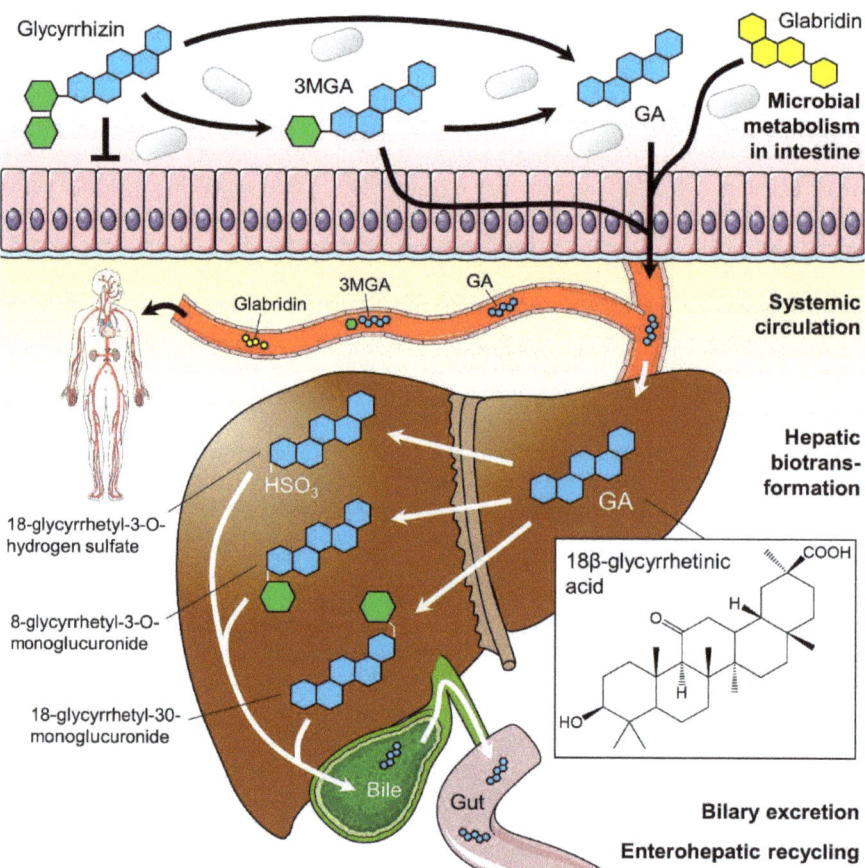

Figure 2. Suggested glycyrrhizin metabolism. Dependent on the gut microbiome glycyrrhizin is stepwise hydrolyzed to 3β-monoglucuronyl-18β-glycyrrhetinic acid (3MGA) and 18β-glycyrrhetinic acid (GA; blue structure) in the intestines. Both 3MGA and GA were absorbed from the gut and transported systemically in the bloodstream. In the liver, they undergo hepatic biotransformation before products were excreted via bile. The flavonoid glabridin (yellow structure) is also absorbed from the gut and circulates in the blood in its aglycone form. The hepatic metabolization of glabridin is not shown here. Green hexagons: glucuronic acid. Parts of the figure were drawn by using pictures from Servier Medical Art (http://smart.servier.com), licensed under a Creative Commons Attribution 3.0 Unported License (https://creativecommons.org/licenses/by/3.0).

The further bioactive constituent, glabridin (Figure 1d), has shown low oral bioavailability in rats. Microsomal studies by Cao et al. [42] demonstrated that glabridin is mainly metabolized by hepatic glucuronidation. They also found that the intestine contributes to glabridin glucuronidation to a much lesser extent. After the intestinal absorption process involving P-glycoprotein, glabridin appears in the human plasma and in the liver as the free (aglycone) form that also circulates within the bloodstream [43,44].

The digestion of licorice is still not completely understood. Interestingly, the bioavailability of glycyrrhizin is reduced when consumed as licorice [45], suggesting that some components of the licorice root may interact with glycyrrhizin during intestinal absorption, reducing its oral bioavailability [46]. Some recent animal studies on rats indicated that there might be further metabolites of GA as causal candidates for the described pharmacological effects [47,48]. In addition, it should be mentioned that the enterohepatic circulation of GA has not yet been studied in humans. However, similar steps can be expected, because GA metabolites can be hydrolyzed by human gastrointestinal bacteria as well [6].

2.2. Pharmacodynamics of Licorice Constituents and Metabolites

Licorice intake induces physiological effects similar to aldosterone and corticosteroids. Resembling steroid-like structures, both 3MGA and GA are able to bind to the mineralocorticoid receptor (MR) in the distal tubules of the kidney (direct effect), although competitive binding assays revealed that the affinities of MR for licorice metabolites were up to 10,000 times weaker than those for adrenocortical hormones [49]. In a normal physiological state, MR is activated by aldosterone to increase sodium and water resorption into the blood and potassium excretion into the urine mediating sodium and water homeostasis within the kidneys. However, it is unclear how the direct effects of 3MGA and GA on MR contribute to the effect of licorice. Although there is some evidence of this direct effect in vitro [50], the relative affinity for MR compared to aldosterone as well as low serum levels of GA after licorice consumption, which did not reach the concentrations necessary to affect aldosterone or cortisol binding to MRs in humans, question that theory [51]. In addition, hyper-mineralocorticosteroid effects were not observed in patients or animals with severe adrenal insufficiency [52]. It is much more likely that metabolites of glycyrrhizin promote a change in cortisol metabolism [53]. Cortisol acts as an agonist for aldosterone to activate MR with equal affinity but circulates in 100–1000-times higher plasma concentrations than that of aldosterone. In adult tissues, the type II isozyme of 11β-hydroxysteroid dehydrogenase (11β-HSD2) is expressed in the distal nephron of the kidney [54], in smooth muscle cells and endothelial cells of the vascular wall [55], in the heart [56] and in the brain [57], where it serves to protect the MR from being overly activated by cortisol [53,58]. 11β-HSD2 converts 'active' cortisol to the 'inactive' cortisone which has a very low affinity for MR. Monder et al. [59] described a strong inhibitory effect of GA for 11β-HSD2 using rat kidney homogenates for in vitro analysis. In addition, oral glycyrrhizin administration inhibited renal 11β-HSD2 activity in rats in a dose-dependent manner [59,60]. Kato et al. [61] suggested that 3MGA, not GA, is the mainly causative agent of licorice-induced pseudohyperaldosteronism. In the kidneys, 11β-HSD2 inhibition by 3MGA or GA (K_i: 5–10 nM) results in a significant increase of active cortisol concentration in the renal tissue leading to a syndrome of apparent mineralocorticoid excess (Figure 3a) [52,62]. In the vascular wall, it increases arterial tone enhancing contractile responses to pressor hormones and reducing endothelial nitric oxide production [57,63]. Further animal studies reported a markedly inhibitory effect of GA on hepatic ring A-reduction of aldosterone by two other hepatic enzymes (5β-reductase and 3β-hydroxysteroid dehydrogenase), increasing the circulating aldosterone levels [64].

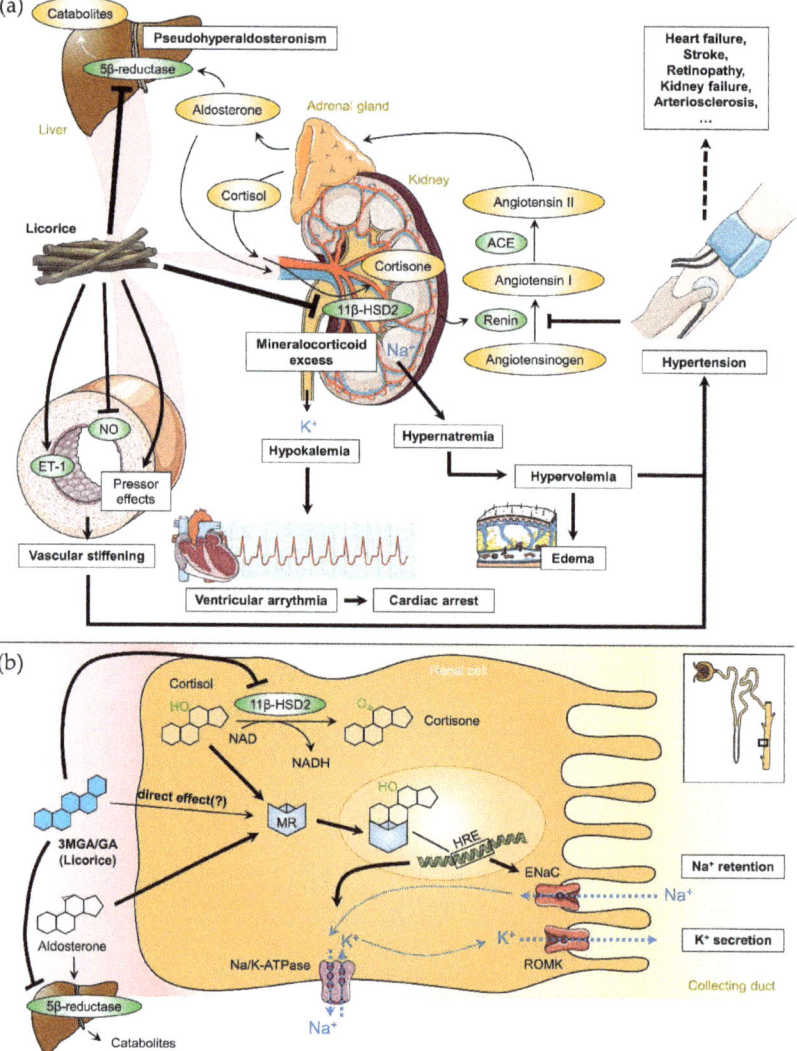

Figure 3. (a) Correlation between licorice intake, the renin-angiotensin-aldosterone-system and licorice-induced adverse effects on the cardiovascular system. (b) Detailed pharmacodynamics of 3β-monoglucuronyl-18β-glycyrrhetinic acid (3MGA) and 18β-glycyrrhetinic acid (GA; blue structure) in the kidney. In addition to a possible direct binding to the mineralocorticoid receptor (MR), 3MGA and GA have inhibiting effects on 11β-hydroxysteroid dehydrogenase type 2 (11β-HSD2) and 5β-reductase. 11β-HSD2 converts cortisol to cortisone; 5β-reductase is involved in the degradation of aldosterone in the liver. Inhibition of both enzymes contributes to apparent mineralocorticoid excess. The insert shows the localization of the processes within the Henle loop. ACE: angiotensin converting enzyme, ENaC: epithelial sodium channel, ET-1: endothelin 1, HRE: hormone response element, NAD(H): nicotinamide adenine dinucleotide, NO: nitric oxide, ROMK: renal outer medullary potassium channel. Parts of the figure were drawn by using pictures from Servier Medical Art (http://smart.servier.com), licensed under a Creative Commons Attribution 3.0 Unported License (https://creativecommons.org/licenses/by/3.0).

A vasorelaxant effect of glabridin was described in rat mesenteric arteries, which was associated with the opening of potassium channels and a concomitant rise in tissue cyclic guanosine monophosphate levels [65].

Taken together, intake of licorice induces a mild form of apparent mineralocorticoid excess causing MRs to be activated by both cortisol and aldosterone via inhibition of enzymes necessary for their catabolism (Figure 3). The direct effects of 3MGA and GA on MRs seem to be only negligible in physiological conditions. In the kidney, MR activation leads to transcription of epithelial sodium channel (ENaC), Na^+/K^+ ATPase and mitochondrial enzymes, which accelerate adenosine triphosphate (ATP)-production (Figure 3b). The final consequences comprise elevated BP, sodium and water retention, decreased plasma potassium (hypokalemia) and caused a suppression of plasma renin and aldosterone levels [66]. In vascular smooth muscle cells, MR activation may further cause vascular stiffening by remodeling of the vascular wall [67]. Furthermore, direct effects of MR activation were described for the rat heart [68].

2.3. Licorice-Induced Hypertension

Licorice mediates its effect on BP primarily via the inhibition of renal 11β-HSD2 by 3MGA and GA (Figure 3a). Water and sodium retention in the kidney increase the blood volume and elevate BP [5]. The body countermeasures with a refractory lowering of the renin secretion in the kidneys, followed by decreased aldosterone production in the adrenal cortex via angiotensin II. However, the increasing level of cortisol (together with unrestricted activation of MR by cortisol) causes pseudohyperaldosteronism. This in turn results in further increasing blood volume and preload of the heart, thereby raising the mean arterial pressure. Furthermore, GA mediates the development of hypertension via decreased bioavailability of NO and activation of the vascular endothelin (ET-1) system (Figure 3a) which was accompanied by impaired endothelium-dependent relaxation in rats [69]. Activation of the endothelin system was also observed in human hypertension [70], and there is some evidence that increased ET-1 may be related to hypertensive end-organ damage and remodeling [71]. Interestingly, an infusion of GA into the rat brain elevated BP without affecting renal sodium and water resorption [72]. This finding indicated a central hypertensinogenic effect of licorice and suggested a more complex regulation of licorice-induced hypertension beyond the inhibition of 11β-HSD2.

Since a correlation between licorice ingestion and BP looks undeniable, further evaluation of quantities is necessary. Leskinen et al. [28] found that a daily intake of 290–370 mg licorice elevated both systolic and diastolic BP after two weeks. Furthermore, an increase of the extracellular fluid volume (hypervolemia) and amplified pressure wave reflection from the peripheral circulation was reported. Hautaniemi et al. [73] demonstrated that in addition to extracellular volume expansion, licorice increased stiffness of large arteries and systemic vascular resistance. A linear dose-response relationship between licorice intake and elevated BP was first proposed by Sigurjónsdóttir et al. [27], who found that a daily ingestion of 75 mg GA (~50 g of licorice) was sufficient to cause a significant increase in systolic BP within a period of two weeks. Similar correlations were later reported by a meta-analysis: analyzing the data of 18 studies (337 patients), systolic and diastolic BP seem to rise dose-dependently suggesting a public recommendation of avoiding excessive licorice consumption [74]. Based on the results of a 12-week experiment with 39 healthy female volunteers, van Gelderen et al. [75] proposed a no-effect level of 2 mg/kg GA per day (equal to 6 g licorice for a person with a body weight of 60 kg).

Two questions remain: 1. Is there any evidence that licorice will increase BP in patients dealing with hypotension? 2. Can general practitioners advocate the complementation of a normal diet with an intake of black licorice or other products containing GA in hypotensive patients? In 1994, it was reported that a 63-year old type 2 diabetic patient was treated for postural hypotension using licorice (3 g of GA/day) as treatment [76]. The patient's BP increased from 90/60 mmHg to 130/80 mmHg in an upright position in 7 days of therapy. Thus, there might be some indications that licorice has its place in clinical therapy, but this must be further investigated in a double-blind, randomized, place-controlled trial to avoid bias.

The case reports of licorice-induced hypertension found in the literature range from mild and reversible forms to severe resistant hypertension requiring hospitalization. In consequence of the elevated BP some patients developed hypertensive encephalopathy or cerebrovascular accidents [77–79]. Acute heart failure, pulmonary edema [80–82] or generalized edema [83–85] can be caused by the sodium retaining effect of licorice (Figure 3a). Interestingly, the occurrence of edema associated with hypertension seems to be characteristic for the 'licorice syndrome'. This is in contrast to true mineralocorticoid excess, where edema is typically absent as a result of the "sodium escape" phenomenon [86,87]. An observed increase in plasma concentration of atrial natriuretic peptide (ANP) after long-term consumption of licorice may be considered a physiological, albeit ineffective, response to prevent fluid retention and development of hypertension [88].

The effects of licorice on aldosterone secretion differ between the genders independently of the BP levels; women seem to be more susceptible to licorice intake [89,90]. A possible explanation for this gender difference are many other hormonal (estrogenic and antiandrogenic) effects exhibited by licorice in addition to its activity via MR. At least the alterations of the calcium metabolism that were observed in healthy women in response to licorice are probably influenced by several further components of the root such as glabridin, which shows estrogen-like activity [89].

There is very rare and controversial information about the correlation between licorice and the development of pulmonary hypertension. A possible contribution of licorice to pulmonary hypertension was suggested by Ruszymah et al. [91] after they had observed an increase in right atrial pressure and thickening of the pulmonary vessels of rats after GA administration. On the other hand, Yang et al. [92] described the attenuation of pulmonary hypertension progression and pulmonary vascular remodeling by glycyrrhizin in a monocrotaline-induced pulmonary hypertension rat model. Here, further studies are needed.

2.3.1. Meta-analyses of Human Trials

In 2017, Penninkilampi et al. [74] reviewed the association between licorice intake, hypertension and hypokalemia. In a broad-based meta-analysis, they confirmed a significant increase in both systolic (5.45 mmHg; 95% confidence interval (CI) 3.51–7.39) and diastolic BP (3.19 mmHg; 95% CI 0.10–6.29) after chronic intake of products containing GA. Since physiological effects are not directly induced by licorice but rather by GA, the GA consumption was calculated for most of the studies. A GA content of 0.2% was approximated for black licorice [74] although the concentration of GA can obviously vary from product to product. Thus, the mean intake of 377.9 mg GA is equal to 189 g of licorice [74] and accounts for the described increase in systolic and diastolic BP. A further meta- and trial sequential analysis by Luis et al. [87] (26 trials, 985 patients) confirmed the significant increase in diastolic BP (1.74 mmHg; 95% CI 0.83–2.62) associated with the hypernatremia caused by licorice consumption. As mentioned by Penninkilampi et al. [74], most of the trials included in their meta-analysis were performed with volunteers. Selection bias in using volunteers and not random participants might be limiting results. The authors found that patients had higher increases in BP after a long intake of GA. They stratified the data in <4 weeks and ≥4 weeks and got elevations of 7.83 mmHg (95% CI 3.69–11.98) and 4.44 mmHg (95% CI 3.20–5.68), respectively. This confirmed the dose-response relationship and a positive correlation between GA dose and changes in both systolic and diastolic BP [74]. The significant increase of 5.45 mmHg might not cause adverse effects in a healthy individual. However, combined with hypokalemia, it can lead to problems in individuals dealing with uncontrolled hypertension [74]. There have been case reports of patients with hypertensive crises where high licorice-intake in combination with hypertension caused hospitalization [93]. Compared with the modest results found in the meta-analysis on the available literature, the number of case reports with serious events or death after chronic licorice ingestion appears excessive [74]. A history of high licorice consumption alone is mostly sufficient to induce a toxic state. The degree of hypokalemia can be severe to cause a lethal arrhythmia [5].

2.3.2. Treatment

In most cases, hypertension and hypervolemia induced by licorice is reversible once intake is stopped. If treatment of licorice-induced hypertension should be necessary, patients will usually be treated as normal hypertensive patients with antihypertensive therapy [94]. Different biochemical analyses will indicate a state of hyperaldosteronism by displaying low plasma potassium and lower levels of plasma renin and aldosterone. Antihypertensive therapy that targets the MR, such as spironolactone, seems to be the primary choice [69]. In rats, it was shown that blocking MR normalized BP [69]. Spironolactone works as a competitive aldosterone antagonist reducing the number of ENaC and Na^+/K^+-ATPase in reverse to aldosterone and cortisol. However, spironolactone treatment is only suggested for an acute hypertensive crisis. Lifestyle interventions should be advised against chronic hypertension caused by high ingestion of licorice and GA-containing products. Depending on the severity, either less ingestion of licorice or a complete stop will be necessary. The ESC guidelines state that grade 2 or 3 hypertension have to be treated with antihypertensive therapy [32]. This accounts for a clinically measured systolic BP ≥ 160 mmHg and/or a diastolic BP ≥ 100 mmHg. Since the effects on electrolyte-levels are delayed, it is furthermore important to stabilize electrolytes, with specific focus of on potassium. When licorice-induced hypertension is treated, it should be kept in mind that it can take up to six months to reverse the mineralocorticoid-like effects of licorice due to its long half-life and the duration required to normalize the renin-angiotensin-aldosterone-system [95].

Indeed, the ESC guidelines for treating hypertension mention that the intake of licorice could influence BP. They address that the medical history should include use of licorice [32]. However, there are no further comments on how licorice-induced hypertension should be treated. An intervention study aimed to investigate whether hypertensive patients were more sensitive to the inhibition of 11β-HSD2 than normotensive patients [96] and found that after 4 weeks of licorice consumption, the mean increase in systolic BP was 3.5 mmHg in healthy individuals and 15.3 mmHg in hypertensive subjects. The mean rise in diastolic BP confirmed this with an increase of 3.6 in mmHg in normotensive and 9.3 mmHg in hypertensive patients. The p-value showed significant differences in both systolic (p = 0.004) and diastolic BP (p = 0.03) [96]. Thus, the authors concluded that subjects with essential hypertension are more sensitive to the licorice-induced inhibition of 11β-HSD2 than normotensive subjects. This finding supports the suggestion that licorice might have stronger adverse effects in patients suffering from hypertension.

However, the available data on this topic is limited and of modest quality and only one clinical trial can be found (Table 1). Further double-blind randomized placebo-controlled studies would be necessary to determine the clinical effects of licorice intake in both healthy and non-healthy individuals.

Table 1. Studies investigating the effects of licorice intake on the human cardiovascular system.

Author (Year), Country	Study Design	n	Drug	Daily Dose	Duration	Relevant Results
Epstein et al. (1977) [97], New Zealand	Pre-post intervention	14	Licorice	100–200 g	1–4 weeks	Serious metabolic effects due to modest licorice intake.
Forslund et al. (1989) [88], Finland	Pre-post intervention	15	Licorice	100 g	8 weeks	Increase in plasma ANP; Decrease in antidiuretic hormone, aldosterone, and plasma renin activity.
MacKenzie et al. (1990) [98], The Netherlands	Pre-post intervention	10	GA	500 mg	8 days	Inhibition of 11β-HSD2.
Kageyama et al. (1992) [99], Japan	Pre-post intervention	58	Glycyrrhizin	225 mg	7 days	Changes in cortisol metabolism.
Bernadini (1994) [100], Italy	Pre-post intervention		Licorice root extract	108-814 mg glycyrrhizin	14 days	Depression of plasma renin activity favored by subclinical disease.
Armanini et al. (1996) [101], Italy	Pre-post intervention	6	Licorice concentrate	7 g (500 mg GA)	7 days	Decreased activity of 11β-HSD2.
van Gelderen et al. (2000) [75], USA	Double-blind randomized controlled	39	GA	0–4 mg per kg	8 weeks	No-effect level: 2 mg/kg GA per day.
Sigurjónsdóttir et al. (2001) [27], Iceland/Sweden	Pre-post intervention	24	Licorice	50–200 g	2–4 weeks	Increase in SBP.
Sigurjónsdóttir et al. (2003) [96], Sweden	Pre-post intervention	25	Licorice	100 g	4 weeks	Increase in SBP and DBP. Subjects with essential hypertension are more sensitive to licorice-induced rise in BP.
Sigurjónsdóttir et al. (2006) [90], Sweden	Pre-post intervention	25	Licorice	100 g	4 weeks	The effect on aldosterone secretion differs between the genders.
Sobieszcyk et al. (2010) [102], USA	Randomized double-blind placebo-controlled crossover	15	GA	130 mg	14 days	Attenuated vasodilatory function on VSMCs.
Tu et al. (2010) [103], China	Two-phase randomized crossover	16	Glycyrrhizin	2 × 150 mg	14 days	Induction of CYP3A.
Yan et al. (2013) [104], China	Two-phase randomized crossover	14	Glycyrrhizin (salt tablet)	3 × 75 mg	6 days	No induction of P-glycoprotein.
Leksinen et al. (2014) [28], Finland ClinicalTrials: NCT01742702	Non-randomized, controlled open label	20	Licorice	290–370 mg glycyrrhizin	14 days	Increase in SBP, DBP, extracellular volume and amplified pressure wave reflection from the periphery.
Hautaniemi et al. (2017) [73], Finland	Non-randomized, controlled open label	22	Licorice	290–370 mg glycyrrhizin	14 days	Increase in SBP, DBP, central pulse pressure, extracellular fluid volume and aortic to popliteal pulse wave velocity.

11β-HSD2: 11-β-hydrogenase type II enzyme; ANP: atrial natriuretic peptide; BP: blood pressure; CYP3A: cytochrome P450 3A4; DBP: diastolic blood pressure; GA: 18β-glycyrrhetinic acid; SBP: systolic blood pressure; VSMC: vascular smooth muscle cell.

2.4. Cardiovascular Effects of Licorice

Licorice traditionally has been prescribed for treatment of cardiovascular disorders, but its effects are not just benign. From the cardiovascular complication described in the literature, cardiac arrhythmias are the most serious side effect caused by licorice intake due to severe hypokalemia (Figure 3a) [105]. The depletion of the body's potassium stores can cause a prolongation of the QT interval, which is closely connected with ventricular arrhythmias and tachycardia [106]. As a consequence, several patients experienced a cardiac arrest with a subsequent recovery [107–109]. Konik et al. [110] described a case of coronary artery spasm induced by licorice. The vasospastic effect of licorice was attributed to changes in endothelin and nitric oxide systems. Recently, a Polish clinical study found a correlation of arterial stiffness parameters with estimated cardiovascular risks in humans [111]. Transient visual loss, migraines and posterior reversible encephalopathy syndrome has also been demonstrated in a few cases. It is assumed that GA inhibits angiogenesis due to inhibition of reactive oxygen species generation [112]. Sobieszcyk et al. [102] found an additional attenuated vascular smooth muscle vasodilatory function without BP changes in healthy humans after 11β-HSD2 inhibition through GA. They proposed that in states of 11β-HSD2 inactivation, non-aldosterone-mediated activation of vascular MRs may contribute to vascular dysfunction and possibly to CVDs.

In rats, cardioprotective effects of licorice and its metabolites were observed, which are mostly related to their antioxidant properties. Thirty days of licorice intake improved cardiac function and preserved histology of cardiomyocytes either by augmentation of endogenous antioxidants or by reduction in oxidative stress. Thus, licorice may delay the progression of ischemic heart disease [113]. Ohja et al. [114] further described a cardioprotective effect against oxidative stress in myocardial ischemia-reperfusion injury after ingestion of *Glycyrrhiza glabra*. Another animal study indicated that GA protects against isoproterenol-induced oxidative stress in rat myocardium decreasing lipid hydroperoxides and isoprostanes and increasing superoxide dismutase and glutathione levels [115].

Some studies suggested that the flavonoid glabridin may also have beneficial effects on the cardiovascular system. The effects described comprise inhibition of low density lipoprotein oxidation and atherogenesis [116], a possible inhibition of NADPH oxidase or an increase in the expression of antioxidant enzymes observed in macrophages [117]. Glabridin also stimulates DNA synthesis in human endothelial cells and demonstrated a bi-phasic proliferative effect on human vascular smooth muscle cells. The combination of an inhibition of smooth muscle cell proliferation and an induction of endothelial cell proliferation may be beneficial for the prevention of atherosclerosis [118,119]. Most recently, Huang et al. [120] reported that glabridin is able to prevent doxycyclin-induced cardiotoxicity in mice through the prevention of gut microbiota dysbiosis. Nevertheless, it remains unclear to which extent these effects contribute to the putative therapeutic actions of licorice.

2.5. Interaction of Licorice with Prescribed Drugs

Licorice can interfere with cardiac medications, e.g., with drugs used in the treatment of hypertension such as angiotensin converting enzyme (ACE)-inhibitors [121]. Some licorice compounds including glabridin and GA can interact with other drugs and the human liver microsomal cytochromes P450 and P450 3A4 (CYP3A4) systems [122–125]. Animal [126,127] and human studies [103] showed that glycyrrhizin has an inductive effect on CYP3A including CYP3A4 and the effect on CYP3A4 may be related to an activation of human pregnane X receptor (hPXR) [103,128]. Other studies described that CYP3A4 was inactivated by licorice extract and glabridin in a time- and concentration-dependent manner [124]. CYP3A4 is involved in the metabolism of xenobiotics [122], roughly half the drugs that are in use today, suggesting that the influence of licorice on CYP3A4 activity needs to be further investigated.

Heck et al. [129] described a toxic effect potentiation of warfarin, a cardiac drug that requires strict dosage adjustment, due to the inhibition of the hepatic microsomal enzymes by licorice.

Matsumoto et al. [130] investigated the effects of licorice on ABC-transporters. Using an in vivo ATPase assay, they demonstrated that licorice root and GA can inhibit P-glycoprotein. A two-phase randomized crossover trial by Yan et al. [104] revealed at least no induction effect on the P-glycoprotein expression after continuous glycyrrhizin administration (225 mg/day) for 6 days. The authors proposed that further research was needed to study the direct inhibition effect of glycyrrhizin on P-glycoprotein. For the pharmaceutical use, it is important to know and consider the interaction between licorice and drugs metabolized by CYP3A4 and P-glycoprotein.

Licorice decreases the bioavailability of cyclosporine and is thus contraindicated [120] in conjunction with this drug [128]. The intake of licorice should be done with caution, when using antihypertensive drugs. ACE-inhibitors, e.g., captopril, inhibit the angiotensin converting enzyme, limiting levels of angiotensin and aldosterone. It was shown that ACE-inhibitors enhance the effects of 11β-HSD2 which may contribute to the natriuretic effect [131]. Hypokalemia is one of the most serious adverse effects of licorice intake and should be completely avoided with loop-diuretics and thiazides since it can lead to serious hypokalemia and hospitalization [132].

The combination of medicine containing licorice and digitalis can cause toxicity, especially in elderly patients. There has been one reported case of digoxin toxicity due to licorice-induced hypokalemia [133].

2.6. Contraindications and Effects of Licorice Overconsumption

Licorice and its derivatives are affirmed as 'Generally Recognized as Safe' (GRAS) for use in foods by the United States Food and Drug Administration (21 CFR 184.1408). Nevertheless, tolerable upper limits of licorice intake have been provided by several institutions: the European Scientific committee of Food recommends that the daily ingestion should not exceed 100 mg of glycyrrhizin (60–70 g of licorice) [134]; the Dutch Nutrition Information Bureau advised against a daily consumption above 200 mg of glycyrrhizin (150 g of licorice) [2]. Since most consumers are not aware of possible health hazards, and there are currently no precise declaration data of glycyrrhizin on food, it is difficult to control licorice intake. Furthermore, it has to be investigated if sporadic intake carries the same risks compared to the daily consumption that is analyzed in most studies. Licorice is found in diet gum, cough mixtures, tea and herbal medicine. Having a mixed intake of these products will accumulate the quantity of GA in vivo, and therefore, increase the risk of symptoms.

In general, people aged over 40, patients with history of cardiac disease or more susceptible to cardiac arrhythmias should avoid excess licorice intake in order to obviate arrhythmias or cardiac arrest caused by licorice-induced hypokalemia. One study investigated patients treated with traditional Japanese medicine containing licorice [135]. They discovered that 24.2% of the patients treated with this medicine developed hypokalemia 34 days after administration. Hypokalemia is a serious state that increases the risk of arrhythmia and is associated with an up to 10-time increase in all-cause mortality [74]. The meta-analysis by Penninkilampi et al. [74] summarized other side effects including rhabdomyolysis, paralysis, hypertensive encephalopathy and cardiac arrest. That is why patients who are on medicines lowering potassium levels (such as thiazide or loop diuretics) should also minimize their licorice intake. The same applies for patients suffering from diarrhea or alcoholism, which can worsen hypokalemia. Licorice can be dangerous in patients treated with antihypertensive drugs such as ACE-inhibitors and diuretics. Due to the salt-retaining effect of 3MGA and GA, people suffering from congestive heart failure or resistant hypertension should completely abstain from products containing licorice. This is also advisable for patients taking digoxin or warfarin to avoid the risk of toxicity. Since 3MGA and GA are known to inhibit 11β-HSD2, licorice ingestion during pregnancy should be avoided. GA consumption impaired the development of the respiratory systems in rats because the conversion of cortisone into cortisol plays an important role in lung maturation [136].

3. Conclusions

In recent years, the mechanisms of action of licorice and its active components have become understood in more detail. The use of licorice in herbal medicine is obviously a result of some positive effects. Hence, it has become one of the most used herbs in traditional Chinese medicine and is still used in China to treat gastric symptoms and respiratory diseases today [10]. Numerous studies have reported about effects of the different compounds found in the licorice root. Glabridin has been proven to be a potent antioxidant with hypoglycemic effects [21]. Referring to studies, glycyrrhizin possesses a wide range of pharmacological effects described as antiulcer and anti-inflammatory [11–13], antiviral [14,15], anticariogenic [137,138] and antispasmodic [139,140].

The utilization of some licorice compounds in a clinical setting is still under investigation. This applies also for artificial GA derivatives such as carbenoxolone [141] or acetoxolone [142]. Glycyrrhizin was identified as an attractive drug candidate for cancer therapy after demonstrating an apoptotic effect on tumor cells [143]. Today, researchers are intensely investigating the applicability of licorice in treatment of breast and prostate cancer. The antitumor activity has attracted the attention of many scientists, since cancer is still one of the leading causes of death in humans around the globe [10].

Nevertheless, due to some safety considerations associated with chronic high-dose intake, licorice should still be consumed with caution. With the elucidation of licorice constituents and the discovery that 3MGA and GA affect the renin-angiotensin-aldosterone-system, pseudohyperaldosteronism is the obvious adverse effect; however, other side effects such as hypertension, hypokalemia and hypernatremia have also been proven. If left untreated, they can cause arrhythmia and, in a worst-case scenario, cardiac arrest. Omar et al. [30,40] have described in detail why licorice should be handled more as medicine than as a candy and that excess licorice consumption can cause serious life-threatening complications, especially in individuals already dealing with high BP and patients under treatment with anti-hypertensive drugs. Adverse effects of high-dose licorice intake have been attributed to glycyrrhizin, 3MGA and GA. Since the final toxicology report has been published in 2007, therapeutic doses of licorice are generally recommended as safe in humans [144]. Especially Scandinavian countries have a higher intake of licorice, and in addition, their licorice has a higher GA concentration [121]. This suggests a need of public focus on the negative effects of licorice on cardiovascular health. However, this is also needed in China, where licorice is widely used in medical practice; here, the knowledge of licorice's interaction with prescription medicines is quite important to avoid possible iatrogenic accidents.

Author Contributions: Conceptualization, M.R.D., D.G. and M.K.; methodology, M.R.D.; validation, D.G., M.W. and M.K.; investigation, M.R.D.; resources, M.I.; data curation, D.G. and M.K.; writing—original draft preparation, M.K., M.R.D. and D.G.; writing—review and editing, M.K., D.G. and M.W.; visualization, M.K.; supervision, D.G.

Funding: This research received no external funding.

Acknowledgments: The authors would like to thank Walter Welß (Botanical Garden of Erlangen) for kindly providing photos of *Glycyrrhiza glabra*.

Conflicts of Interest: The authors declare no conflict of interest.

Abbreviations

11β-HSD2	11-β-hydrogenase type II enzyme
3MGA	3β-monoglucuronyl-18β-glycyrrhetinic acid
ACE	Angiotensin converting enzyme
ANP	Atrial natriuretic peptide
ATP	Adenosine triphosphate
BP	Blood pressure
CI	Confidence interval
CVD	Cardiovascular disease
CYP3A4	Cytochrome P450 3A4
DBP	Diastolic blood pressure
ENaC	Epithelial sodium channel
ESC	European Society of Cardiology
ET-1	Endothelin 1
GA	18β-glycyrrhetinic acid
HRE	Hormone response element
MR	Mineralocorticoid receptor
NAD(H)	Nicotinamide adenine dinucleotide
NO	Nitric oxide
ROMK	Renal outer medullary potassium channel
SBP	Systolic blood pressure
VSMC	Vascular smooth muscle cell

References

1. Foster, C.A.; Church, K.S.; Poddar, M.; Van Uum, S.H.; Spaic, T. Licorice-induced hypertension: A case of pseudohyperaldosteronism due to jelly bean ingestion. *Postgrad. Med.* **2017**, *129*, 3293–3331. [CrossRef] [PubMed]
2. Fenwick, G.R.; Lutomski, J.; Nieman, C. Liquorice, Glycyrrhiza glabra L.—Composition, uses and analysis. *Food Chem.* **1990**, *38*, 1191–1243. [CrossRef]
3. Kao, T.C.; Wu, C.H.; Yen, G.C. Bioactivity and potential health benefits of licorice. *J. Agric. Food Chem.* **2014**, *62*, 542–553. [CrossRef] [PubMed]
4. Fiore, C.; Eisenhut, M.; Ragazzi, E.; Zanchin, G.; Armanini, D. A history of the therapeutic use of liquorice in europe. *J. Ethnopharmacol.* **2005**, *99*, 317–324. [CrossRef]
5. Allcock, E.; Cowdery, J. Hypertension induced by liquorice tea. *BMJ Case Rep.* **2015**. [CrossRef]
6. Isbrucker, R.A.; Burdock, G.A. Risk and safety assessment on the consumption of licorice root (Glycyrrhiza sp.), its extract and powder as a food ingredient, with emphasis on the pharmacology and toxicology of glycyrrhizin. *Regul. Toxicol. Pharmacol.* **2006**, *46*, 167–192. [CrossRef]
7. NCCIH. Licorice Root. Available online: http://nccih.nih.gov/health/licoriceroot (accessed on 24 September 2019).
8. Sabbadin, C.; Bordin, L.; Donà, G.; Manso, J.; Avruscio, G.; Armanini, D. Licorice: From pseudohyperaldosteronism to therapeutic uses. *Front. Endocrinol.* **2019**. [CrossRef]
9. Volqvartz, T.; Vestergaard, A.L.; Aagaard, S.K.; Andreasen, M.F.; Lesnikova, I.; Uldbjerg, N.; Larsen, A.; Bor, P. Use of alternative medicine, ginger and licorice among Danish pregnant women—A prospective cohort study. *BMC Complement. Altern. Med.* **2019**, *19*, 5. [CrossRef]
10. Yang, R.; Wang, L.Q.; Yuan, B.C.; Liu, Y. The pharmacological activities of licorice. *Planta Med.* **2015**, *81*, 1654–1669. [CrossRef]
11. Aly, A.M.; Al-Alousi, L.; Salem, H.A. Licorice: A possible anti-inflammatory and anti-ulcer drug. *AAPS PharmSciTech* **2005**, *6*, E74–E82. [CrossRef]
12. Jalilzadeh-Amin, G.; Najarnezhad, V.; Anassori, E.; Mostafavi, M.; Keshipour, H. Antiulcer properties of Glycyrrhiza glabra L. Extract on experimental models of gastric ulcer in mice. *Iranian J. Pharm. Res.* **2015**, *14*, 1163–1170.
13. Yang, R.; Yuan, B.C.; Ma, Y.S.; Zhou, S.; Liu, Y. The anti-inflammatory activity of licorice, a widely used chinese herb. *Pharm. Biol.* **2017**, *55*, 5–18. [CrossRef] [PubMed]
14. Wang, L.; Yang, R.; Yuan, B.; Liu, Y.; Liu, C. The antiviral and antimicrobial activities of licorice, a widely-used Chinese herb. *Acta Pharm. Sin. B* **2015**, *5*, 310–315. [CrossRef] [PubMed]
15. Fukuchi, K.; Okudaira, N.; Adachi, K.; Odai-Ide, R.; Watanabe, S.; Ohno, H.; Yamamoto, M.; Kanamoto, T.; Terakubo, S.; Nakashima, H.; et al. Antiviral and antitumor activity of licorice root extracts. *In Vivo* **2016**, *30*, 777–785. [CrossRef]
16. Huo, H.Z.; Wang, B.; Liang, Y.K.; Bao, Y.Y.; Gu, Y. Hepatoprotective and antioxidant effects of licorice extract against CCl_4-induced oxidative damage in rats. *Int. J. Mol. Sci.* **2011**, *12*, 6529–6543. [CrossRef]
17. Jung, J.-C.; Lee, Y.-H.; Kim, S.H.; Kim, K.-J.; Kim, K.-M.; Oh, S.; Jung, Y.-S. Hepatoprotective effect of licorice, the root of Glycyrrhiza uralensis Fischer, in alcohol-induced fatty liver disease. *BMC Complement. Altern. Med.* **2016**, *16*, 19. [CrossRef]
18. Wang, Z.Y.; Nixon, D.W. Licorice and cancer. *Nutr. Cancer* **2001**, *39*, 1–11. [CrossRef]
19. Rahnama, M.; Mehrabani, D.; Japoni, S.; Edjtehadi, M.; Saberi Firoozi, M. The healing effect of licorice (Glycyrrhiza glabra) on Helicobacter pylori infected peptic ulcers. *J. Res. Med. Sci.* **2013**, *18*, 532–533.
20. Momeni, A.; Rahimian, G.; Kiasi, A.; Amiri, M.; Kheiri, S. Effect of licorice versus bismuth on eradication of Helicobacter pylori in patients with peptic ulcer disease. *Pharmacogn. Res.* **2014**, *6*, 341–344. [CrossRef]
21. Wu, F.; Jin, Z.; Jin, J. Hypoglycemic effects of glabridin, a polyphenolic flavonoid from licorice, in an animal model of diabetes mellitus. *Mol. Med. Rep.* **2013**, *7*, 1278–1282. [CrossRef]
22. Simmler, C.; Pauli, G.F.; Chen, S.N. Phytochemistry and biological properties of glabridin. *Fitoterapia* **2013**, *90*, 160–184. [CrossRef] [PubMed]

23. Stepien, M.; Kujawska-Luczak, M.; Szulinska, M.; Kregielska-Narozna, M.; Skrypnik, D.; Suliburska, J.; Skrypnik, K.; Regula, J.; Bogdanski, P. Beneficial dose-independent influence of *Camellia sinensis* supplementation on lipid profile, glycemia, and insulin resistance in an NaCl-induced hypertensive rat model. *J. Physiol. Pharmacol.* **2018**. [CrossRef]
24. Sontia, B.; Mooney, J.; Gaudet, L.; Touyz, R.M. Pseudohyperaldosteronism, liquorice, and hypertension. *J. Clin. Hypertens.* **2008**, *10*, 153–157. [CrossRef]
25. Varma, R.; Ross, C.N. Liquorice: A root cause of secondary hypertension. *JRSM Open* **2017**, *8*, 2054270416685208. [CrossRef] [PubMed]
26. Morris, D.J. Liquorice: New insights into mineralocorticoid and glucocorticoid hypertension. *R. I. Med.* **1993**, *76*, 251–254.
27. Sigurjónsdóttir, H.Á.; Franzson, L.; Manhem, K.; Ragnarsson, J.; Sigurdsson, G.; Wallerstedt, S. Liquorice-induced rise in blood pressure: A linear dose-response relationship. *J. Hum. Hypertens.* **2001**, *15*, 549–552. [CrossRef]
28. Leskinen, M.H.; Hautaniemi, E.J.; Tahvanainen, A.M.; Koskela, J.K.; Päällysaho, M.; Tikkakoski, A.J.; Kähönen, M.; Kööbi, T.; Niemelä, O.; Mustonen, J.; et al. Daily liquorice consumption for two weeks increases augmentation index and central systolic and diastolic blood pressure. *PLoS ONE* **2014**, *9*, e105607. [CrossRef]
29. Falet, J.P.; Elkrief, A.; Green, L. Hypertensive emergency induced by licorice tea. *CMAJ* **2019**, *191*, E581–E583. [CrossRef]
30. Omar, H.R. The cardiovascular complications of licorice. *Cardiovasc. Endocrinol.* **2013**, *2*, 46–49. [CrossRef]
31. Forouzanfar, M.H.; Liu, P.; Roth, G.A.; Ng, M.; Biryukov, S.; Marczak, L.; Alexander, L.; Estep, K.; Hassen Abate, K.; Akinyemiju, T.F.; et al. Global burden of hypertension and systolic blood pressure of at least 110 to 115 mm hg, 1990–2015. *JAMA* **2017**, *317*, 165–182. [CrossRef]
32. Williams, B.; Mancia, G.; Spiering, W.; Agabiti Rosei, E.; Azizi, M.; Burnier, M.; Clement, D.L.; Coca, A.; de Simone, G.; Dominiczak, A.; et al. 2018 esc/esh guidelines for the management of arterial hypertension. *Eur. Heart J.* **2018**, *39*, 3021–3104. [CrossRef] [PubMed]
33. Charles, L.; Triscott, J.; Dobbs, B. Secondary hypertension: Discovering the underlying cause. *Am. Fam. Phys.* **2017**, *96*, 453–461.
34. Wang, Q.; Qian, Y.; Wang, Q.; Yang, Y.F.; Ji, S.; Song, W.; Qiao, X.; Guo, D.A.; Liang, H.; Ye, M. Metabolites identification of bioactive licorice compounds in rats. *J. Pharm. Biomed. Anal.* **2015**, *115*, 515–522. [CrossRef] [PubMed]
35. Nieman, C. Licorice. *Adv. Food Res.* **1957**, *7*, 339–381.
36. Kim, D.-H.; Lee, S.-W.; Han, M.J. Biotransformation of glycyrrhizin to 18β-glycyrrhetinic acid-3-o-β-d-glucuronide by streptococcus lj-22, a human intestinal bacterium. *Biol. Pharm. Bull.* **1999**, *22*, 320–322. [CrossRef]
37. Hattori, M.; Sakamoto, T.; Yamagishi, T.; Sakamoto, K.; Konishi, K.; Kobashi, K.; Namba, T. Metabolism of glycyrrhizin by human intestinal flora. Ii. Isolation and characterization of human intestinal bacteria capable of metabolizing glycyrrhizin and related compounds. *Chem. Pharm Bull.* **1985**, *33*, 210–217. [CrossRef]
38. Armanini, D.; Nacamulli, D.; Francini-Pesenti, F.; Battagin, G.; Ragazzi, E.; Fiore, C. Glycyrrhetinic acid, the active principle of licorice, can reduce the thickness of subcutaneous thigh fat through topical application. *Steroids* **2005**, *70*, 538–542. [CrossRef]
39. Feng, X.; Ding, L.; Qiu, F. Potential drug interactions associated with glycyrrhizin and glycyrrhetinic acid. *Drug Metab. Rev.* **2015**, *47*, 229–238. [CrossRef]
40. Omar, H.R.; Komarova, I.; El-Ghonemi, M.; Fathy, A.; Rashad, R.; Abdelmalak, H.D.; Yerramadha, M.R.; Ali, Y.; Helal, E.; Camporesi, E.M. Licorice abuse: Time to send a warning message. *Ther. Adv. Endocrinol.* **2012**, *3*, 125–138. [CrossRef]
41. Ploeger, B.; Mensinga, T.; Sips, A.; Meulenbelt, J.; DeJongh, J. A human physiologically-based model for glycyrrhzic acid, a compound subject to presystemic metabolism and enterohepatic cycling. *Pharm. Res.* **2000**, *17*, 1516–1525. [CrossRef]
42. Cao, J.; Chen, X.; Liang, J.; Yu, X.Q.; Xu, A.L.; Chan, E.; Wei, D.; Huang, M.; Wen, J.Y.; Yu, X.Y.; et al. Role of p-glycoprotein in the intestinal absorption of glabridin, an active flavonoid from the root of glycyrrhiza glabra. *Drug Metab. Dispos.* **2007**, *35*, 539–553. [CrossRef]

43. Ito, C.; Oi, N.; Hashimoto, T.; Nakabayashi, H.; Aoki, F.; Tominaga, Y.; Yokota, S.; Hosoe, K.; Kanazawa, K. Absorption of dietary licorice isoflavan glabridin in blood circulation in rats. *J. Nutr. Sci. Vitaminol.* **2007**, *53*, 358–365. [CrossRef]
44. Aoki, F.; Nakagawa, K.; Tanaka, A.; Matsuzaki, K.; Arai, N.; Mae, T. Determination of glabridin in human plasma by solid-phase extraction and lc-ms/ms. *J. Chromatogr. B Analyt. Technol. Biomed. Life Sci.* **2005**, *828*, 70–74. [CrossRef] [PubMed]
45. Raggi, M.A.; Maffei, F.; Bugamelli, F.; Cantelli Forti, G. Bioavailability of glycyrrhizin and licorice extract in rat and human plasma as detected by a hplc method. *Pharmazie* **1994**, *49*, 269–272.
46. Cantelli-Forti, G.; Maffei, F.; Hrelia, P.; Bugamelli, F.; Bernardi, M.; D'Intino, P.; Maranesi, M.; Raggi, M.A. Interaction of licorice on glycyrrhizin pharmacokinetics. *Environ. Health Perspect.* **1994**, *102* (Suppl. 9), 65–68. [CrossRef]
47. Ishiuchi, K.; Morinaga, O.; Ohkita, T.; Tian, C.; Hirasawa, A.; Mitamura, M.; Maki, Y.; Kondo, T.; Yasujima, T.; Yuasa, H.; et al. 18beta-glycyrrhetyl-3-o-sulfate would be a causative agent of licorice-induced pseudoaldosteronism. *Sci. Rep.* **2019**, *9*, 1587. [CrossRef]
48. Morinaga, O.; Ishiuchi, K.; Ohkita, T.; Tian, C.; Hirasawa, A.; Mitamura, M.; Maki, Y.; Yasujima, T.; Yuasa, H.; Makino, T. Isolation of a novel glycyrrhizin metabolite as a causal candidate compound for pseudoaldosteronism. *Sci. Rep.* **2018**, *8*, 15568. [CrossRef]
49. Armanini, D.; Karbowiak, I.; Funder, J.W. Affinity of liquorice derivatives for mineralocorticoid and glucocorticoid receptors. *Clin. Endocrinol.* **1983**, *19*, 609–612. [CrossRef] [PubMed]
50. Calo, L.A.; Zaghetto, F.; Pagnin, E.; Davis, P.A.; De Mozzi, P.; Sartorato, P.; Martire, G.; Fiore, C.; Armanini, D. Effect of aldosterone and glycyrrhetinic acid on the protein expression of pai-1 and p22(phox) in human mononuclear leukocytes. *J. Clin. Endocrinol. Metab.* **2004**, *89*, 1973–1976. [CrossRef]
51. Størmer, F.C.; Reistad, R.; Alexander, J. Glycyrrhizic acid in liquorice—Evaluation of health hazard. *Food Chem. Toxicol.* **1993**, *31*, 303–312. [CrossRef]
52. Stewart, P.M.; Wallace, A.M.; Valentino, R.; Burt, D.; Shackleton, C.H.; Edwards, C.R. Mineralocorticoid activity of liquorice: 11-beta-hydroxysteroid dehydrogenase deficiency comes of age. *Lancet* **1987**, *2*, 821–824. [CrossRef]
53. Ferrari, P. The role of 11beta-hydroxysteroid dehydrogenase type 2 in human hypertension. *Biochim. Biophys. Acta* **2010**, *1802*, 1178–1187. [CrossRef] [PubMed]
54. Atanasov, A.G.; Ignatova, I.D.; Nashev, L.G.; Dick, B.; Ferrari, P.; Frey, F.J.; Odermatt, A. Impaired protein stability of 11beta-hydroxysteroid dehydrogenase type 2: A novel mechanism of apparent mineralocorticoid excess. *J. Am. Soc. Nephrol.* **2007**, *18*, 1262–1270. [CrossRef] [PubMed]
55. Christy, C.; Hadoke, P.W.; Paterson, J.M.; Mullins, J.J.; Seckl, J.R.; Walker, B.R. 11beta-hydroxysteroid dehydrogenase type 2 in mouse aorta: Localization and influence on response to glucocorticoids. *Hypertension* **2003**, *42*, 580–587. [CrossRef]
56. Lombes, M.; Alfaidy, N.; Eugene, E.; Lessana, A.; Farman, N.; Bonvalet, J.P. Prerequisite for cardiac aldosterone action. Mineralocorticoid receptor and 11 beta-hydroxysteroid dehydrogenase in the human heart. *Circulation* **1995**, *92*, 175–182. [CrossRef] [PubMed]
57. Hadoke, P.W.; Christy, C.; Kotelevtsev, Y.V.; Williams, B.C.; Kenyon, C.J.; Seckl, J.R.; Mullins, J.J.; Walker, B.R. Endothelial cell dysfunction in mice after transgenic knockout of type 2, but not type 1, 11beta-hydroxysteroid dehydrogenase. *Circulation* **2001**, *104*, 2832–2837. [CrossRef]
58. Van Uum, S.H. Liquorice and hypertension. *Neth. J. Med.* **2005**, *63*, 119–120.
59. Monder, C.; Stewart, P.M.; Lakshmi, V.; Valentino, R.; Burt, D.; Edwards, C.R. Licorice inhibits corticosteroid 11 beta-dehydrogenase of rat kidney and liver: In vivo and in vitro studies. *Endocrinology* **1989**, *125*, 1046–1053. [CrossRef]
60. Tanahashi, T.; Mune, T.; Morita, H.; Tanahashi, H.; Isomura, Y.; Suwa, T.; Daido, H.; Gomez-Sanchez, C.E.; Yasuda, K. Glycyrrhizic acid suppresses type 2 11 beta-hydroxysteroid dehydrogenase expression in vivo. *J. Steroid Biochem. Mol. Biol.* **2002**, *80*, 441–447. [CrossRef]
61. Kato, H.; Kanaoka, M.; Yano, S.; Kobayashi, M. 3-monoglucuronyl-glycyrrhetinic acid is a major metabolite that causes licorice-induced pseudoaldosteronism. *J. Clin. Endocrinol. Metab.* **1995**, *80*, 1929–1933. [CrossRef]
62. Hammer, F.; Stewart, P.M. Cortisol metabolism in hypertension. *Best Pract. Res. Clin. Endocrinol. Metab.* **2006**, *20*, 337–353. [CrossRef] [PubMed]

63. Souness, G.W.; Brem, A.S.; Morris, D.J. 11 beta-hydroxysteroid dehydrogenase antisense affects vascular contractile response and glucocorticoid metabolism. *Steroids* **2002**, *67*, 195–201. [CrossRef]
64. Latif, S.A.; Conca, T.J.; Morris, D.J. The effects of the licorice derivative, glycyrrhetinic acid, on hepatic 3α- and 3β-hydroxysteroid dehydrogenases and 5α- and 5β-reductase pathways of metabolism of aldosterone in male rats. *Steroids* **1990**, *55*, 52–58. [CrossRef]
65. Chanda, D.; Prieto-Lloret, J.; Singh, A.; Iqbal, H.; Yadav, P.; Snetkov, V.; Aaronson, P.I. Glabridin-induced vasorelaxation: Evidence for a role of bkca channels and cyclic gmp. *Life Sci.* **2016**, *165*, 26–34. [CrossRef] [PubMed]
66. Farese, R.V., Jr.; Biglieri, E.G.; Shackleton, C.H.; Irony, I.; Gomez-Fontes, R. Licorice-induced hypermineralocorticoidism. *N. Engl. J. Med.* **1991**, *325*, 1223–1227. [CrossRef]
67. Tarjus, A.; Amador, C.; Michea, L.; Jaisser, F. Vascular mineralocorticoid receptor and blood pressure regulation. *Curr. Opin. Pharmacol.* **2015**, *21*, 138–144. [CrossRef]
68. Ohtake, M.; Hattori, T.; Murase, T.; Takahashi, K.; Takatsu, M.; Ohtake, M.; Miyachi, M.; Watanabe, S.; Cheng, X.W.; Murohara, T.; et al. Glucocorticoids activate cardiac mineralocorticoid receptors in adrenalectomized dahl salt-sensitive rats. *Nagoya J. Med. Sci.* **2014**, *76*, 59–72.
69. Quaschning, T.; Ruschitzka, F.; Shaw, S.; Luscher, T.F. Aldosterone receptor antagonism normalizes vascular function in liquorice-induced hypertension. *Hypertension* **2001**, *37*, 801–805. [CrossRef]
70. Schiffrin, E.L.; Deng, L.Y.; Sventek, P.; Day, R. Enhanced expression of endothelin-1 gene in resistance arteries in severe human essential hypertension. *J. Hypertens.* **1997**, *15*, 57–63. [CrossRef]
71. Ergul, S.; Parish, D.C.; Puett, D.; Ergul, A. Racial differences in plasma endothelin-1 concentrations in individuals with essential hypertension. *Hypertension* **1996**, *28*, 652–655. [CrossRef]
72. Gomez-Sanchez, E.P.; Gomez-Sanchez, C.E. Central hypertensinogenic effects of glycyrrhizic acid and carbenoxolone. *Am. J. Physiol.* **1992**, *263*, E1125–E1130. [CrossRef] [PubMed]
73. Hautaniemi, E.J.; Tahvanainen, A.M.; Koskela, J.K.; Tikkakoski, A.J.; Kähönen, M.; Uitto, M.; Sipilä, K.; Niemelä, O.; Mustonen, J.; Pörsti, I.H. Voluntary liquorice ingestion increases blood pressure via increased volume load, elevated peripheral arterial resistance, and decreased aortic compliance. *Sci. Rep.* **2017**, *7*, 10947. [CrossRef] [PubMed]
74. Penninkilampi, R.; Eslick, E.M.; Eslick, G.D. The association between consistent licorice ingestion, hypertension and hypokalaemia: A systematic review and meta-analysis. *J. Hum. Hypertens.* **2017**, *31*, 699–707. [CrossRef] [PubMed]
75. Van Gelderen, C.E.; Bijlsma, J.A.; van Dokkum, W.; Savelkoul, T.J. Glycyrrhizic acid: The assessment of a no effect level. *Hum. Exp. Toxicol.* **2000**, *19*, 434–439. [CrossRef]
76. Basso, A.; Dalla Paola, L.; Erle, G.; Boscaro, M.; Armanini, D. Licorice ameliorates postural hypotension caused by diabetic autonomic neuropathy. *Diabetes Care* **1994**, *17*, 1356. [CrossRef]
77. Van der Zwan, A. Hypertension encephalopathy after liquorice ingestion. *Clin. Neurol. Neurosurg.* **1993**, *95*, 35–37. [CrossRef]
78. Russo, S.; Mastropasqua, M.; Mosetti, M.A.; Persegani, C.; Paggi, A. Low doses of liquorice can induce hypertension encephalopathy. *Am. J. Nephrol.* **2000**, *20*, 145–148. [CrossRef]
79. Bramont, C.; Lestradet, C.; Godart, L.; Faivre, R.; Narboni, G. cerebral vascular accident caused by alcohol-free licorice. *Presse Med.* **1985**, *14*, 746.
80. Chamberlain, J.J.; Abolnik, I.Z. Pulmonary edema following a licorice binge. *West J. Med.* **1997**, *167*, 184–185.
81. Chamberlain, T.J. Licorice poisoning, pseudoaldosteronism, and heart failure. *JAMA* **1970**, *213*, 1343. [CrossRef]
82. Hasegawa, J.; Suyama, Y.; Kinugawa, T.; Morisawa, T.; Kishimoto, Y. Echocardiographic findings of the heart resembling dilated cardiomyopathy during hypokalemic myopathy due to licorice-induced pseudoaldosteronism. *Cardiovasc. Drugs Ther.* **1998**, *12*, 599–600. [CrossRef] [PubMed]
83. Sailler, L.; Juchet, H.; Ollier, S.; Nicodeme, R.; Arlet, P. generalized edema caused by licorice: A new syndrome. Apropos of 3 cases. *Rev. Med. Interne* **1993**, *14*, 984. [CrossRef]
84. Johns, C. Glycyrrhizic acid toxicity caused by consumption of licorice candy cigars. *CJEM* **2009**, *11*, 94–96. [CrossRef] [PubMed]
85. Francini-Pesenti, F.; Puato, M.; Piccoli, A.; Brocadello, F. Liquorice-induced hypokalaemia and water retention in the absence of hypertension. *Phytother. Res.* **2008**, *22*, 563–565. [CrossRef] [PubMed]

86. Negro, A.; Rossi, E.; Regolisti, G.; Perazzoli, F. Liquorice-induced sodium retention. Merely an acquired condition of apparent mineralocorticoid excess? A case report. *Ann. Ital. Med. Int.* **2000**, *15*, 296–300.
87. Luis, A.; Domingues, F.; Pereira, L. Metabolic changes after licorice consumption: A systematic review with meta-analysis and trial sequential analysis of clinical trials. *Phytomedicine* **2018**, *39*, 17–24. [CrossRef]
88. Forslund, T.; Fyhrquist, F.; Froseth, B.; Tikkanen, I. Effects of licorice on plasma atrial natriuretic peptide in healthy volunteers. *J. Intern. Med.* **1989**, *225*, 95–99. [CrossRef]
89. Mattarello, M.J.; Benedini, S.; Fiore, C.; Camozzi, V.; Sartorato, P.; Luisetto, G.; Armanini, D. Effect of licorice on PTH levels in healthy women. *Steroids* **2006**, *71*, 403–408. [CrossRef]
90. Sigurjonsdottir, H.A.; Axelson, M.; Johannsson, G.; Manhem, K.; Nyström, E.; Wallerstedt, S. The liquorice effect on the RAAS differs between the genders. *Blood Press* **2006**, *15*, 169–172. [CrossRef]
91. Ruszymah, B.H.; Nabishah, B.M.; Aminuddin, S.; Khalid, B.A. Effects of glycyrrhizic acid on right atrial pressure and pulmonary vasculature in rats. *Clin. Exp. Hypertens.* **1995**, *17*, 575–591. [CrossRef]
92. Yang, P.-S.; Kim, D.-H.; Lee, Y.J.; Lee, S.-E.; Kang, W.J.; Chang, H.-J.; Shin, J.-S. Glycyrrhizin, inhibitor of high mobility group box-1, attenuates monocrotaline-induced pulmonary hypertension and vascular remodeling in rats. *Respir. Res.* **2014**, *15*, 148. [CrossRef] [PubMed]
93. Ottenbacher, R.; Blehm, J. An unusual case of licorice-induced hypertensive crisis. *S. D. Med.* **2015**, *68*, 346–347. [PubMed]
94. Schulze zur Wiesch, C.; Sauer, N.; Aberle, J. hypertension and hypokalemia—A reninoma as the cause of suspected liquorice-induced arterial hypertension. *Dtsch. Med. Wochenschr.* **2011**, *136*, 882–884. [CrossRef] [PubMed]
95. Epstein, M.T.; Espiner, E.A.; Donald, R.A.; Hughes, H. Liquorice toxicity and the renin-angiotensin-aldosterone axis in man. *BMJ* **1977**, *1*, 209–210. [CrossRef] [PubMed]
96. Sigurjonsdottir, H.A.; Manhem, K.; Axelson, M.; Wallerstedt, S. Subjects with essential hypertension are more sensitive to the inhibition of 11 beta-hsd by liquorice. *J. Hum. Hypertens.* **2003**, *17*, 125–131. [CrossRef] [PubMed]
97. Epstein, M.T.; Espiner, E.A.; Donald, R.A.; Hughes, H. Effect of eating liquorice on the renin-angiotensin aldosterone axis in normal subjects. *Br. Med. J.* **1977**, *1*, 488–490. [CrossRef]
98. MacKenzie, M.A.; Hoefnagels, W.H.; Jansen, R.W.; Benraad, T.J.; Kloppenborg, P.W. The influence of glycyrrhetinic acid on plasma cortisol and cortisone in healthy young volunteers. *J. Clin. Endocrinol. Metab.* **1990**, *70*, 1637–1643. [CrossRef]
99. Kageyama, Y.; Suzuki, H.; Saruta, T. Glycyrrhizin induces mineralocorticoid activity through alterations in cortisol metabolism in the human kidney. *J. Endocrinol.* **1992**, *135*, 147–152. [CrossRef]
100. Bernardi, M.; D'Intino, P.E.; Trevisani, F.; Cantelli-Forti, G.; Raggi, M.A.; Turchetto, E.; Gasbarrini, G. Effects of prolonged ingestion of graded doses of licorice by healthy volunteers. *Life Sci.* **1994**, *55*, 863–872. [CrossRef]
101. Armanini, D.; Lewicka, S.; Pratesi, C.; Scali, M.; Zennaro, M.C.; Zovato, S.; Gottardo, C.; Simoncini, M.; Spigariol, A.; Zampollo, V. Further studies on the mechanism of the mineralocorticoid action of licorice in humans. *J. Endocrinol. Invest.* **1996**, *19*, 624–629. [CrossRef]
102. Sobieszczyk, P.; Borlaug, B.A.; Gornik, H.L.; Knauft, W.D.; Beckman, J.A. Glycyrrhetinic acid attenuates vascular smooth muscle vasodilatory function in healthy humans. *Clin. Sci.* **2010**, *119*, 437–442. [CrossRef] [PubMed]
103. Tu, J.H.; He, Y.J.; Chen, Y.; Fan, L.; Zhang, W.; Tan, Z.R.; Huang, Y.F.; Guo, D.; Hu, D.L.; Wang, D.; et al. Effect of glycyrrhizin on the activity of cyp3a enzyme in humans. *Eur. J. Clin. Pharmacol.* **2010**, *66*, 805–810. [CrossRef] [PubMed]
104. Yan, M.; Fang, P.-F.; Li, H.-D.; Xu, P.; Liu, Y.-P.; Wang, F.; Cai, H.-L.; Tan, Q.-Y. Lack of effect of continuous glycyrrhizin administration on the pharmacokinetics of the p-glycoprotein substrate talinolol in healthy volunteers. *Eur. J. Clin. Pharmacol.* **2013**, *69*, 515–521. [CrossRef] [PubMed]
105. Bocker, D.; Breithardt, G. induction of arrhythmia by licorice abuse. *Z. Kardiol.* **1991**, *80*, 389–391. [PubMed]
106. Eriksson, J.W.; Carlberg, B.; Hillorn, V. Life-threatening ventricular tachycardia due to liquorice-induced hypokalaemia. *J. Intern. Med.* **1999**, *245*, 307–310. [CrossRef] [PubMed]
107. Bannister, B.; Ginsburg, R.; Shneerson, J. Cardiac arrest due to liquorice induced hypokalaemia. *BMJ* **1977**, *2*, 738–739. [CrossRef]
108. Crean, A.M.; Abdel-Rahman, S.E.; Greenwood, J.P. A sweet tooth as the root cause of cardiac arrest. *Can. J. Cardiol.* **2009**, *25*, e357–e358. [CrossRef]

109. Campana, A.; Manzo, M.; Brigante, M.; Marrazzo, N.; Melchiorre, G. an unusual cause of cardiac arrest. *Ital. Heart J. Suppl.* **2003**, *4*, 510–513.
110. Konik, E.; Kurtz, E.G.; Sam, F.; Sawyer, D. Coronary artery spasm, hypertension, hypokalemia and licorice. *J. Clin. Case Rep.* **2012**, *2*, 143. [CrossRef]
111. Tąpolska, M.; Spałek, M.; Szybowicz, U.; Domin, R.; Owsik, K.; Sochacka, K.; Skrypnik, D.; Bogdański, P.; Owecki, M. Arterial Stiffness Parameters Correlate with Estimated Cardiovascular Risk in Humans: A Clinical Study. *Int. J. Environ. Res. Public Health* **2019**, *16*, 2547. [CrossRef]
112. Banerjee, A.; Giri, R. Chapter 9—Nutraceuticals in gastrointestinal disorders. In *Nutraceuticals*; Gupta, R.C., Ed.; Academic Press: Boston, MA, USA, 2016; pp. 109–122.
113. Ojha, S.K.; Sharma, C.; Golechha, M.J.; Bhatia, J.; Kumari, S.; Arya, D.S. Licorice treatment prevents oxidative stress, restores cardiac function, and salvages myocardium in rat model of myocardial injury. *Toxicol. Ind. Health* **2015**, *31*, 140–152. [CrossRef] [PubMed]
114. Ojha, S.; Golechha, M.; Kumari, S.; Bhatia, J.; Arya, D.S. Glycyrrhiza glabra protects from myocardial ischemia–reperfusion injury by improving hemodynamic, biochemical, histopathological and ventricular function. *Exp. Toxicol. Pathol.* **2013**, *65*, 219–227. [CrossRef] [PubMed]
115. Haleagrahara, N.; Varkkey, J.; Chakravarthi, S. Cardioprotective effects of glycyrrhizic acid against isoproterenol-induced myocardial ischemia in rats. *Int. J. Mol. Sci.* **2011**, *12*, 7100–7113. [CrossRef] [PubMed]
116. Fuhrman, B.; Buch, S.; Vaya, J.; Belinky, P.A.; Coleman, R.; Hayek, T.; Aviram, M. Licorice extract and its major polyphenol glabridin protect low-density lipoprotein against lipid peroxidation: In vitro and ex vivo studies in humans and in atherosclerotic apolipoprotein e-deficient mice. *Am. J. Clin. Nutr.* **1997**, *66*, 267–275. [CrossRef] [PubMed]
117. Rosenblat, M.; Belinky, P.; Vaya, J.; Levy, R.; Hayek, T.; Coleman, R.; Merchav, S.; Aviram, M. Macrophage enrichment with the isoflavan glabridin inhibits nadph oxidase-induced cell-mediated oxidation of low density lipoprotein. A possible role for protein kinase C. *J. Biol. Chem.* **1999**, *274*, 13790–13799. [CrossRef]
118. Somjen, D.; Knoll, E.; Vaya, J.; Stern, N.; Tamir, S. Estrogen-like activity of licorice root constituents: Glabridin and glabrene, in vascular tissues in vitro and in vivo. *J. Steroid Biochem. Mol. Biol.* **2004**, *91*, 147–155. [CrossRef]
119. Somjen, D.; Kohen, F.; Jaffe, A.; Amir-Zaltsman, Y.; Knoll, E.; Stern, N. Effects of gonadal steroids and their antagonists on DNA synthesis in human vascular cells. *Hypertension* **1998**, *32*, 39–45. [CrossRef]
120. Huang, K.; Liu, Y.; Tang, H.; Qiu, M.; Li, C.; Duan, C.; Wang, C.; Yang, J.; Zhou, X. Glabridin prevents doxorubicin-induced cardiotoxicity through gut microbiota modulation and colonic macrophage polarization in mice. *Front. Pharmacol.* **2019**. [CrossRef]
121. Meyer, R. Pseudohyperaldosteronismus: Lakritzverzehr mit Folgen. *Dtsch. Arztebl. Int.* **2000**, *97*, A-596.
122. Wang, X.; Zhang, H.; Chen, L.; Shan, L.; Fan, G.; Gao, X. Liquorice, a unique "guide drug" of traditional chinese medicine: A review of its role in drug interactions. *J. Ethnopharmacol.* **2013**, *150*, 781–790. [CrossRef]
123. Tsukamoto, S.; Aburatani, M.; Yoshida, T.; Yamashita, Y.; El-Beih, A.A.; Ohta, T. Cyp3a4 inhibitors isolated from licorice. *Biol. Pharm Bull.* **2005**, *28*, 2000–2002. [CrossRef] [PubMed]
124. Kent, U.M.; Aviram, M.; Rosenblat, M.; Hollenberg, P.F. The licorice root derived isoflavan glabridin inhibits the activities of human cytochrome p450s 3a4, 2b6, and 2c9. *Drug Metab. Dispos.* **2002**, *30*, 709–715. [CrossRef] [PubMed]
125. Lv, Q.L.; Wang, G.H.; Chen, S.H.; Hu, L.; Zhang, X.; Ying, G.; Qin, C.Z.; Zhou, H.H. In vitro and in vivo inhibitory effects of glycyrrhetinic acid in mice and human cytochrome p450 3a4. *Int. J. Environ. Res. Public Health* **2015**, *13*, 84. [CrossRef] [PubMed]
126. Paolini, M.; Barillari, J.; Broccoli, M.; Pozzetti, L.; Perocco, P.; Cantelli-Forti, G. Effect of liquorice and glycyrrhizin on rat liver carcinogen metabolizing enzymes. *Cancer Lett.* **1999**, *145*, 35–42. [CrossRef]
127. Paolini, M.; Pozzetti, L.; Sapone, A.; Cantelli-Forti, G. Effect of licorice and glycyrrhizin on murine liver cyp-dependent monooxygenases. *Life Sci.* **1998**, *62*, 571–582. [CrossRef]
128. Hou, Y.C.; Lin, S.P.; Chao, P.D. Liquorice reduced cyclosporine bioavailability by activating p-glycoprotein and cyp 3a. *Food Chem.* **2012**, *135*, 2307–2312. [CrossRef]
129. Heck, A.M.; DeWitt, B.A.; Lukes, A.L. Potential interactions between alternative therapies and warfarin. *Am. J. Health Syst. Pharm.* **2000**, *57*, 1221–1227, quiz 1228–1230. [CrossRef]

130. Matsumoto, T.; Kaifuchi, N.; Mizuhara, Y.; Warabi, E.; Watanabe, J. Use of a caco-2 permeability assay to evaluate the effects of several kampo medicines on the drug transporter p-glycoprotein. *J. Nat. Med.* **2018**, *72*, 897–904. [CrossRef]
131. Kerstens, M.N.; Dullaart, R.P. 11 beta-hydroxysteroid-dehydrogenase: Characteristics and the clinical significance of a key enzyme in cortisol metabolism. *Ned. Tijdschr. Geneeskd.* **1999**, *143*, 509–514.
132. Buhl, L.F.; Pedersen, F.N.; Andersen, M.S.; Glintborg, D. Licorice-induced apparent mineralocorticoid excess compounded by excessive use of terbutaline and high water intake. *BMJ Case Rep.* **2018**. [CrossRef]
133. Harada, T.; Ohtaki, E.; Misu, K.; Sumiyoshi, T.; Hosoda, S. Congestive heart failure caused by digitalis toxicity in an elderly man taking a licorice-containing chinese herbal laxative. *Cardiology* **2002**, *98*, 218. [CrossRef] [PubMed]
134. Scientific Committee on Food. *Opinion of the Scientific Committee on Food on Glycyrrhizinic acid and Its Ammonium Salt*; Scientific Committee on Food: Brussels, Belgium, 2003.
135. Shimada, S.; Arai, T.; Tamaoka, A.; Homma, M. Liquorice-induced hypokalaemia in patients treated with yokukansan preparations: Identification of the risk factors in a retrospective cohort study. *BMJ Open* **2017**, *7*, e014218. [CrossRef] [PubMed]
136. Nazari, S.; Rameshrad, M.; Hosseinzadeh, H. Toxicological effects of Glycyrrhiza glabra (licorice): A review. *Phytother. Res.* **2017**, *31*, 1635–1650. [CrossRef]
137. Steinberg, D.; Sgan-Cohen, H.D.; Stabholz, A.; Pizanty, S.; Segal, R.; Sela, M.N. The anticariogenic activity of glycyrrhizin: Preliminary clinical trials. *Isr. J. Dent. Sci.* **1989**, *2*, 153–157. [PubMed]
138. Segal, R.; Pisanty, S.; Wormser, R.; Azaz, E.; Sela, M.N. Anticariogenic activity of licorice and glycyrrhizine i: Inhibition of in vitro plaque formation by streptococcus mutans. *J. Pharm. Sci.* **1985**, *74*, 79–81. [CrossRef] [PubMed]
139. Jia, J.; Li, Y.; Lei, Z.; Hao, Y.; Wu, Y.; Zhao, Q.; Wang, H.; Ma, L.; Liu, J.; Zhao, C.; et al. Relaxative effect of core licorice aqueous extract on mouse isolated uterine horns. *Pharm. Biol.* **2013**, *51*, 744–748. [CrossRef]
140. Yang, L.; Chai, C.Z.; Yan, Y.; Duan, Y.D.; Henz, A.; Zhang, B.L.; Backlund, A.; Yu, B.Y. Spasmolytic mechanism of aqueous licorice extract on oxytocin-induced uterine contraction through inhibiting the phosphorylation of heat shock protein 27. *Molecules* **2017**, *22*, 1392. [CrossRef]
141. Peskar, B.M. Effect of carbenoxolone on prostaglandin synthesizing and metabolizing enzymes and correlation with gastric mucosal carbenoxolone concentrations. *Scand. J. Gastroenterol. Suppl.* **1980**, *65*, 109–114.
142. Wang, L.J.; Geng, C.A.; Ma, Y.B.; Huang, X.Y.; Luo, J.; Chen, H.; Zhang, X.M.; Chen, J.J. Synthesis, biological evaluation and structure-activity relationships of glycyrrhetinic acid derivatives as novel anti-hepatitis b virus agents. *Bioorg. Med. Chem. Lett.* **2012**, *22*, 3473–3479. [CrossRef]
143. Hibasami, H.; Iwase, H.; Yoshioka, K.; Takahashi, H. Glycyrrhizin induces apoptosis in human stomach cancer kato iii and human promyelotic leukemia hl-60 cells. *Int. J. Mol. Med.* **2005**, *16*, 233–236. [CrossRef]
144. Asl, M.N.; Hosseinzadeh, H. Review of pharmacological effects of *Glycyrrhiza* sp. And its bioactive compounds. *Phytother. Res.* **2008**, *22*, 709–724. [CrossRef] [PubMed]

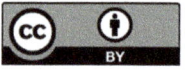

© 2019 by the authors. Licensee MDPI, Basel, Switzerland. This article is an open access article distributed under the terms and conditions of the Creative Commons Attribution (CC BY) license (http://creativecommons.org/licenses/by/4.0/).

MDPI
St. Alban-Anlage 66
4052 Basel
Switzerland
Tel. +41 61 683 77 34
Fax +41 61 302 89 18
www.mdpi.com

Foods Editorial Office
E-mail: foods@mdpi.com
www.mdpi.com/journal/foods

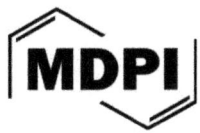

www.ingramcontent.com/pod-product-compliance
Lightning Source LLC
LaVergne TN
LVHW070542100526
838202LV00012B/355